The CHILI PEPPER DIET

The CHILI PEPPER DIET

The Natural Way to

Control Cravings,
Boost Metabolism
and Lose Weight

Heidi Allison

Health Communications, Inc.
Deerfield Beach, Florida

www.hci-online.com

Library of Congress Cataloging-in-Publication Data

Allison, Heidi.
    The chili pepper diet : the natural way to control cravings, boost metabolism, and lose weight / Heidi Allison.
       p.   cm.
    Includes bibliographical references.
    ISBN 1-55874-926-8 (tradepaper)
1. Cookery (Hot peppers) 2. Hot peppers. I. Title.

TX803.P46 A43 2002
641.6'384—dc21

2002023686

Publisher: Health Communications, Inc.
               3201 S.W. 15th Street
               Deerfield Beach, FL 33442-8190

Cover design by Lisa Camp
Inside book design by Lawna Patterson Oldfield
Inside book formatting by Dawn Von Strolley Grove
Chili pepper photo styling by Heidi Allison

This book is dedicated to my family.

CONTENTS

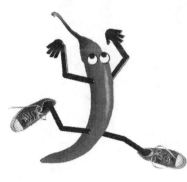

Acknowledgments ix

Introduction: God's Little Miracle xi

Part One: Body Chemistry and Dieting

1. Why Diets Fail 3
2. The Chili Connection 13

Part Two: The Chili Pepper Diet

3. Use Flavor—Not Fat 43
4. Not All Chilies Are Created Equal 69
5. Chilies: All the Way from Hot to Mild 87
6. The Chili Pepper Diet 113
7. Smart Choices 181
8. Restaurant Rules 215

Part Three: The Chili Pepper Diet
       Recipes for Success

9. Hot and Healthy Recipes 243
   Breadspreads, 245 • Egg Dishes, 253
   Vegetarian Dishes, 259 • Salad Dressings, 269

Poultry Dishes, 279 • Seafood, 287 • Sides and Salads, 301 • Meat, 313
Soups, 319 • Pasta, 331 • Marinades and Sauces, 339 • Salsas, 347
Seasoning Blends, 363 • Desserts, 371

Where to Find Chili Products 377
Bibliography 379
Index 393

ACKNOWLEDGMENTS

My deepest gratitude to the incredible staff at HCI: Peter Vegso for believing in this book, Christine Belleris, Allison Janse and Erica Orloff for their editing expertise and unwavering support, Larissa Hise Henoch for her enthusiasm and guidance with the chili pepper photographs, Lawna Oldfield for skilled text layout and design, Lisa Camp for the marvelous cover design, Anthony Clausi and "Uncle Joe" Kerman for their proofreading, Dawn Grove for her typesetting, and Peter Quintal for scanning.

I would like to thank my agent, David Robie, for his insight, guidance and support throughout this project.

To everyone who participated in the

Chili Pepper Diet Study—I learned so much from all your experiences. You were my inspiration and muse.

I owe a debt of gratitude to everyone who participated in the Chili Pepper Diet study. Your enthusiasm, dedication and commitment were my inspiration and muse. A special thanks to Justin Pierce, Chef Jamie Shannon, Margaret Farrell, M.S., Lena Ting, M.S., Ami Spitalnick, Dr. Carol Jong, Michael Yarish, Dr. Alan Hirsch, Danise Coon, Dr. Julie Menella, Dr. Marci Pelchat, Dr. Hyman Gross, Dr. Keith Sharkey, Dr. Peter Blumberg, Barton Wright and Susan Green.

GOD'S LITTLE MIRACLE

Thirteen years ago I was dying—physically, emotionally and spiritually. At thirty-two, I had a cholesterol count of 256 mg/dl, was ninety pounds overweight and miserable. Food controlled my life—I obsessed about it, dreamed about it, worried about it and cried about it. Every day was a struggle (that I lost) to control my addiction to food. Until I discovered chilies.

I never had a serious weight problem until I became pregnant. Within days of conception, uncontrollable cravings for ice cream, cheeseburgers and French fries emerged. And my metabolism had changed. It seemed every morsel of food that passed my lips turned to fat—quickly. By the time I had missed my first cycle, I had gained thirty pounds. By the second trimester, I was tipping the scales at sixty pounds gained. At delivery, I was close to two hundred pounds.

I thought the weight would drop off after my son was born, but it didn't. My mother sent exercise videos and coupons for Lean Cuisine. Girlfriends enrolled me in aerobics classes, and my husband hired a personal trainer to help me burn off the fat. None of these efforts worked.

I coped by denying I had a problem. I continued to wear my oversized maternity clothes eighteen months after delivery, convincing myself that my metabolism just needed more time to revert to its prepregnancy state. My wake-up call came one day in the market when a cashier asked me, "When is your baby due?" I was so ashamed, I wanted to crawl out the door.

Feeling depressed, I tried several diets to lose weight. I struggled at Weight Watchers for three months without losing a pound. The portion sizes never seemed enough, which gnawed at my stomach and my morale. Feeling hungry and deprived was slow torture, and I abandoned the diet.

The Pritikin plan seemed like the answer to my prayers. Unfortunately, it wasn't. This program promised weight loss without hunger through eating carbohydrates. However, the food tasted like cardboard, and substituting those carbohydrates for the fat packed another twelve pounds on my frame within two months.

Neither were low-carbohydrate diets the answer to painless weight loss. Not only did I feel nauseated on this regimen, but living without fruit, bread and pasta proved too difficult to sustain. Three weeks into the diet I felt so deprived I could have killed for a bagel.

Depression turned to desperation, and I started smoking cigarettes to lose weight. Although I had gone through agony quitting ten years before, I rationalized I'd quit as soon as I lost weight. Within one month, I was smoking a pack a day and hadn't lost an ounce.

I hit rock bottom when my doctor bluntly told me I should know the answer with my medical background—"Losing weight is easy if you just stop stuffing your mouth." First I cried, then I got really angry. What an arrogant statement—obviously she had never struggled with the uncontrollable urges that compelled me to eat. What I needed was a way to control my appetite, not a patronizing lecture. I turned to God and prayed, "Please help me find a way." At my lowest point in this struggle with my weight, an inner-strength and determination began to surface. I decided to devise my own diet.

I started to analyze different cultures where obesity wasn't a national problem, such as Japan and indigenous cultures in Latin America. Obviously something was working in these cuisines. A primary characteristic of these foods was a low fat content in tandem with different flavoring agents including chilies. As I substituted soy sauces, spices, vinegars and chilies for the fat, my enjoyment for low-fat foods increased while my fat cravings decreased for the first time in two years. Within two weeks of eating this sublime-tasting low-fat food, I could put my fork down after eating half a plate of food without feeling deprived.

This was remarkable since most dieters will tell you it takes months to lose cravings for fats and sweets on conventional low-fat diets. For others, those cravings never subside. Something in this diet was facilitating this process. As I experimented more with chilies, I started to crave spicy food. I just couldn't eat a meal without chilies. So, I focused on what my body was really telling me when it craved fat and sugar—eating fat and sugar gave me a sense of calm. They were an easy-to-get over-the-counter "tranquilizer" that took the edge off a hard day. That pint of ice cream, not carrots, made me feel less stressed.

A bit of self-searching brought memories that even as a child, I wanted salami or cream cheese and jam on my bagel, while my brother went for Rice Chex and fruit. It was no coincidence that even then I had definite food preferences, and salty/fats or sweet/fats were my "drugs of choice." Some biochemical factor had to be at work here.

I started researching to look for an answer. I discovered studies linking obesity to low levels of endorphins and neurotransmitters, and that eating sweet and fatty foods elevated these chemicals. My intuition was proving right—overeating was not a lack of willpower but rather self-medicating with foods to correct these biochemical imbalances.

I was convinced I had the "why's," now I needed the "what's"— what chemical in chilies decreased my appetite? So, this is where I began my research that eventually lead me to scientists, databases, deep into Peru and even to the Hopi Reservation in Arizona.

My first insight came when I hosted a dinner for a group of physicians while working in the pharmaceutical business. We all ordered Cajun-style blackened catfish. Within minutes, I was sweating and my heart was racing. Knowing these were signs of increased metabolic rate, I turned to my manager and asked if any pharmaceutical company had studied the metabolic effects of "hot foods"? "Yes," he said. "The pharmaceutical industry has been looking into the chemical in chilies for years. It's called capsaicin. Apparently, it has some profound effects on physiology, but we haven't taken it any further. It's available over the counter, and our company feels there's no profit margin in it."

Back into the libraries and databases I went. There I found ongoing studies looking into the effects of capsaicin on animals. When it was used, pain relief, weight loss, cholesterol reduction and other health benefits occurred.

I had found the key I was looking for.

I added chilies, in various forms and amounts, to all my foods and the pounds melted off. Just as nicotine patches took the edge off cigarette withdrawals, *chilies took the angst out of dieting.* I knew I could maintain this diet because it was so easy—no hunger, deprivation, nervousness or fatigue had to be endured. And the food I created had such flavor, I never had the desire to cheat with rich sauces or sweet desserts.

The most amazing discovery I made was that chilies affected my moods—I felt calm and happy on this diet. I was better able to handle the daily stresses that cropped up without anger or fatigue. Even my sleep patterns changed for the better: I woke up after eight hours (instead of five) feeling more rested than I had in years. Chilies were God's little miracle that made a low-fat diet work.

I lost weight in all the right places. My stomach, thighs, hips and upper arms slimmed down, but my face never became haggard. In fact, friends commented that my coloring had taken a rosy glow rather than that stressed pallor most dieters wear. People were noticing a wonderful change and wanted to know "my secret."

Within a year, I was back to my prepregnancy weight and fitting into my size-six jeans. My cholesterol dropped from 256 to 160 with an impressive TC/HDL ratio of 2.5. However, the biggest surprise was my lowered blood pressure. It had always run 120/80, regardless of whether I was fat or thin. Now it routinely measured 90/70, what you'd expect to see in an athlete. Something in chilies was lowering my blood pressure, and it clearly wasn't a consequence of weight loss.

After maintaining this program for six years, I contacted an internist and a registered dietitian. They agreed to assist me in a clinical study to test the program on a larger scale. The clinical study lasted twelve months, and the results showed that chilies *dramatically* enhanced the effects of a low-fat diet. Weight loss increased tenfold! Chilies also countered the negative effects a low-fat diet on cholesterol levels. Unless you get lots of exercise, or lose weight (or both), low-fat diets can actually *increase* your risk for heart disease by decreasing HDL levels (the good kind) and increasing triglyceride levels. Most Americans on low-fat diets do neither. Finally, a chili-spiked low-fat diet lowered high blood pressure levels as effectively as some prescription drugs, while high blood sugar levels plummeted.

This study validated my own unofficial findings. The chili pepper diet helped me get my weight under control and gave me my life back. Now I'd like to share the miracle of chili peppers with you. Join me on this journey as you learn a healthy and tasty new way to eat.

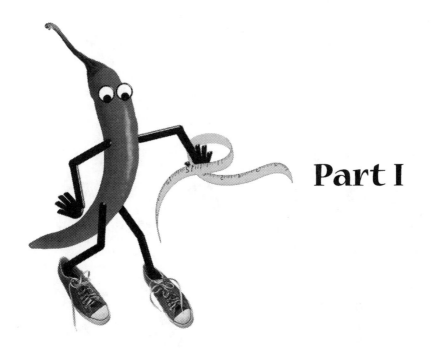

Part I

BODY
CHEMISTRY
AND DIETING

CHAPTER ONE

WHY DIETS FAIL

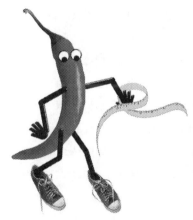

Being fat is becoming America's number-one health problem—over half of us want to lose weight and a third of us need to. The risk of developing high blood pressure, heart disease, diabetes or cancer dramatically rises if you're obese. And if you figure in gallbladder, digestive and pulmonary diseases, being overweight is a serious health problem. With all the abundant information and methods available for weight reduction, why have diets notoriously failed?

In the 1950s, people dieted by counting calories: You cut down on the *amount* of food you ate to lose weight. The theory was that if you dropped 500 calories a day you would lose a pound of fat per week. This sounded great on paper, but it didn't work. This diet made you feel hungry and deprived, and it took the dedication of a martyr to follow. Those who did manage to adhere to the regimen ended up losing muscle instead of fat and simply lowered their metabolism.

During the 1970s, you lost weight by reducing the *type* of food you ate—carbohydrates. Known as ketogenic, this diet claimed that to burn fat you needed to keep your fat and protein intake high. Although these programs promised you wouldn't feel hungry, its "no pain did not equal gain" approach to living without bread, pasta and fruit left most people feeling deprived. The high-fat content of the diet also jacked up cholesterol levels and much of the weight loss proved to be water—not fat.

By the 1980s, dieters were counting fat grams instead. The theory was that fat calories converted to body fat more readily than calories from proteins and carbohydrates; to lose weight you needed to keep the fat intake low and the carbohydrate intake high. According to Kelly Brownwell, a specialist in eating disorders at Yale University, "Our food is lower in fat, but we aren't. If anything, the incidence of obesity has risen." From 1977 to 1996, our fat consumption has decreased 17.5 percent, but obesity has increased 25 percent. If it were that easy to lose weight by cutting down on fat, fewer diets would end in depression and failure.

Another popular diet idea was espoused by several national diet programs, which recommend reducing fat content to 20 to 25 percent to lose weight. The American Heart Association's Diet advocated reducing your fat intake to 30 percent. Unfortunately, the long-term success rate for these types of diets is low. Many people abandon the diet within three years, and regain the weight they lost.

Obviously, low-fat diets are flawed. For this type of diet to work, you need to keep portion sizes small and get lots of exercise. Trouble is, most Americans on low-fat diets do neither. People wind up feeling hungry and deprived, which is stressful, and they abandon the diet. I felt nervous, irritable and fatigued. Others experience sleep disturbances or trouble concentrating at work. But the worst side effect of this type of diet is depression. Even though you desperately want to or even need to lose weight, a low-fat diet is just too difficult to maintain.

To make low-fat dieting bearable, many dieters resort to appetite suppressants. The problem is most of these products are only effective on a short-term basis, if at all, and there are significant side effects to these drugs, such as addiction, increased blood pressure and heart palpitations.

The reason many people can't limit their fats is because they affect us like drugs. In fact, fat cravings are linked to the same physiological mechanism that is responsible for addiction. According to Joseph Piscatella, author of *Controlling Your Fat Tooth*, fats are craved as drugs because they release endorphins, your body's natural painkillers that make you feel good. Other researchers have uncovered that low levels of dopamine, a common substance in the brain, are linked to obesity. It appears a deficit of dopamine triggers fat cravings and increases appetite.

What about diets recommending that fat be reduced to 7 to 10 percent of daily calories? These diets have the advantage that people lose weight quickly and dramatically. But not permanently. Most people who try this type of program drop out. I lasted two months, which is about the average.

This was not an easy diet to follow! My family hated the flavorless food on this diet, and I couldn't convince anyone to become low-fat vegetarians. So, I had to cook separate meals. The extra time it required—from shopping to cooking to cleaning up—just wasn't worth the effort.

As for eating out—think "nightmare." Even in nutrition-crazed

Los Angeles, only two restaurants served nonfat vegetarian-style food, and it was awful. And I dreaded visiting friends for dinner, and I'm sure my friends dreaded my visits just as much. Either it meant extra work for them to accommodate my needs, or they felt guilty I couldn't eat. All in all, this diet didn't fit into the "real world" and was too difficult to maintain.

But the worst part about this "diet" was I *gained* twelve pounds on it! Substituting carbohydrates for the fat didn't work. I felt hungry all the time and compensated by eating vast amounts of carbohydrates to feel "full." Despite the fact I was eating every two hours, I never felt satisfied. By mid-afternoon, I was so tired all I wanted to do was sleep.

Research backs up the futility of very low-fat dieting. Researchers have concluded that obese people need twice the amount of fat as those of normal weight to feel "full." When they go on a low-fat diet, this group compensates by eating large amounts of carbohydrates to feel satisfied. But, carbohydrate calories still count!

Currently, dietitians are focusing not only on fat grams, but also portion sizes to facilitate weight loss. There is a misconception that fat-free means you have carte blanche to eat large portions—it doesn't. Many people have gained weight on a fat-free diets. The truth is, 3,500 calories, whether they are from carbohydrates, proteins or fats, add one pound to your frame.

What about new protein advocates Barry Sears, Ph.D., author of *The Zone*, and Drs. Michael and Mary Eades, authors of *Protein Power*, who stress the solution to treating obesity and heart disease is lowering your insulin levels by restricting carbohydrates. Fat levels of 30 to 45 percent of daily calories in tandem with high levels of protein are advocated to blunt appetite and regulate the hormonal responses responsible for keeping your weight, cholesterol, blood sugar and blood pressure in check.

However, many dietary experts state these programs work because they are merely low in calories. According to Alice Lichtenstein, D.Sc., a researcher at Tufts University, "High protein diets are based on pure science—science fiction that is. If you crunch the numbers, this type of diet works because of caloric restriction—they give a mere 800 to 1,200 calories a day. These diets have also increased cholesterol levels because they endorse high amounts of saturated fats."

Yet the most incriminating opinion comes from the Stanford University researcher, Gerald Raven, M.D., whose studies on insulin resistance were cited by Sears and Eades as the cornerstone of their programs. He states there isn't a shred of evidence to support their claims that insulin resistance is what makes most people gain weight: "This has not been proven, and they have no right to make that claim."

Beyond their sketchy research, high-protein diets have nutritional negatives. These programs have complications such as nausea, ketosis, electrolyte loss, dehydration, constipation, calcium depletion and kidney problems. They also tend to be deficient in fiber, vitamins, minerals and phytochemicals—all nutritional powerhouses that fight heart disease and cancer.

FINDING WHAT WORKED

The diet that worked for me contained a moderate level of fat—a level I could comfortably live on without gorging on carbohydrates to feel "full." It was a nutritionally balanced diet that provided a variety of foods—chicken, fish, lean meats, nonfat and low-fat dairy products, grains, fruits, vegetables and healing oils. Although I wasn't hungry, I did feel deprived because the food tasted like cardboard. I missed the sensual qualities that make dining one of life's greatest pleasures—texture and flavor. This sent me on my chili quest.

According to researchers, flavor is critical for maintaining long-term weight loss. In a three-year study involving 894 patients, researcher A. Kristal and his colleagues concluded that avoiding fats as a flavoring agent was the greatest factor in sustaining weight loss. These researchers uncovered that using margarine on bread and potatoes and avoiding high-fat salad dressing were the hardest habits to keep.

Traditionally, cuisine in America is not only cooked in fat but flavored with fat. I began to look to other cuisines for an answer. Asian food uses different soy sauces and rice wine vinegar. Indian cuisine uses spices such as ginger, mustard seed, turmeric and cumin. Mexican food uses cilantro and chilies. I started to incorporate these ingredients, and the foods I created satisfied both my body and my soul.

I discovered that the more chilies I added to food, the more I liked this cuisine. Low-fat food not only tasted better with chilies, but I was satisfied eating smaller portions. Finally, I could put my fork down after eating half a plate of food without feeling deprived. As an experiment, I started to add chilies to every meal, and the weight started to come off with little effort.

Chilies are the missing link that make a low-fat diet work. The active ingredient in chilies, capsaicin, reduces hunger by activating the neuronal pathways that send signals to the brain that you're "full" but without expanding your waistline, making you feel sluggish, increasing your cholesterol or elevating blood pressure levels.

Chilies convert your body from a fat-storing to a fat-burning mode by releasing neurotransmitters that boost metabolism. Several studies have shown that peppers elevate your metabolic rate for up to five hours after you eat a spicy meal. A study conducted by C. Henry, et. al, found that chili peppers increased metabolic rate by 25 percent. In a Japanese study, researchers found that red pepper both increased metabolism and curbed appetite in men and women. These results are supported by another study published in the *European Journal of Clinical Nutrition*, which found that hot red peppers dramatically increased metabolism.

Other studies have uncovered that chilies affect the regulation of two enzymes involved in fat metabolism that release fat from your fat cells so they can be used as fuel. I had finally found the key I was looking for—a magic ingredient I could add to food that burned fat instead of making me fat.

Moreover, you won't have to endure the stress most low-fat diets create because capsaicin releases endorphins and serotonin, which act to take the angst out of losing weight. Chilies engender a blissful calm while preventing depression as the pounds melt away—without the negative side effects associated with pharmaceutical drugs.

Aside from the tremendous weight-reducing benefits of chilies, these incredible fruits provide protection against degenerative diseases such as cancer, heart disease, stroke, hypertension, ulcers and diabetes, to name a few. Additionally, chilies increase your sexual functioning by activating the nerves involved in the regulation of blood flow to the sexual organs. No other diet promises that!

The indigenous peoples of North and South America call these fruits a "sacred plant," Christopher Columbus called them "red gold." We know them as chilies. They are the key to permanent weight loss and good health!

Sacred Seeds

Although many books have discussed the history of chilies in Latin American cultures, little has been written about the use of chilies in our nature cultures. The Hopi have lived in the United States longer than any other people—they are the original inhabitants of this land. And according to many other Native Americans, the Hopi are also the most spiritual and possess a greater knowledge of healing.

The Hopi live in villages perched on 600-foot desert cliffs in Northern Arizona. It is a stark yet majestically serene landscape—peppered with alkali flats, sage and red-rock canyons. This land is brutally harsh—at night, temperatures drop below freezing, while the scorching summer heat soars over 100°F. Rain is sporadic, at best. A meager 8 to 10 inches fall in this arid land per year. Yet, the Hopi have prevailed in spite of these adverse conditions, largely through their religious beliefs and ceremonies.

What Are Kachina Dolls?

The Hopi believe that all things created by God have spirit or energy—even rocks. Kachina dolls, or *tihu*, are small carved wooden figures that symbolize the spirit of an animal, insect, bird, plant, object, person or spiritual being. Each kachina has a specific function, and the Hopi believe these spiritual beings teach them how to bring rain, heal illness and offer spiritual gratitude.

Although kachinas are referred to as "dolls," they are not toys. These carved figures are believed to contain the power of the kachina, and are treated with respect. To protect the *tihu* from harm, they are hung from beams or on walls in the home. Kachinas are also "fed" cornmeal—often a bowl of

white cornmeal is left near a
kachina, or white cornmeal is
sprinkled near a kachina, which
symbolically feeds its spirit.
To the Hopi, a kachina doll is
much more than an image—a
personal relationship is formed
between the spirit it represents
and the recipient. And it is a
mutually beneficial relationship.
Kachinas act as intermediaries
between the spirit world and the
material world, and intervene
for the Hopi on their behalf. I
was told that the kachina doll
will "speak" to you—it will not
only teach you things but also

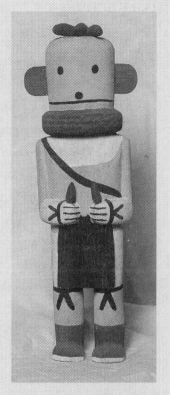

protect you. In a sense, kachinas act as guardian angels
and are considered friends.

Since Hopi men have a higher level of contact with the
spiritual realm, kachina dolls are carved by men and given
to women. Often, they are given as gifts to uninitiated
young girls during the Powamuya (Bean Dance), which is
held in February and the Niman Dance (Home Dance)
that takes place in July. *Tihu* are treasured, and help teach
these young girls about their religion and culture.

Tsil Kachina

Chilies (Tsili) are an important part of Hopi Indian life—they provide nourishment, serve as a medicine and have religious significance.

A Tsili (chili) kachina is a Wawash (runner) kachina, and is characterized by large eyes, ears and chilies. A chili kachina also appears to be a map of where chilies work their magic in the body. Two chilies rest on the abdomen. Capsaicin exerts its effects in the liver and the pancreas located in this area. Three chilies sit on top of the head. Recently, scientists uncovered that three areas in the brain contain a high density of nerves that respond to capsaicin because they have the capsaicin (vanilloid) receptor. These regions regulate appetite (medial basal hypothalamus), body temperature (pre-optic-anterior hypothalamus) and feelings of pleasure through the dopamine pathways (locus ceruleus). Moreover, five chilies appear on the kachina—five chilies were the magic nunber that reduced appetite and promoted health benefits in the Chili Pepper Diet Study.

It is by chance a chili kachina is depicted as a runner? I don't think so. The effects of capsaicin parallel those produced by running. Research has shown that capsaicin triggers the body to burn fat, ups metabolism, increases oxygen consumption rate, reduces appetite, lowers blood pressure, improves sugar metabolism and prompts the body to release endorphins. In many ways, the chili kachina captures the essence of the healing power of this sacred plant.

CHAPTER TWO

THE CHILI CONNECTION

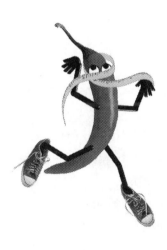

During the last decade, over fifty-eight hundred research studies have investigated the effects of the fiery chemical found in chilies, capsaicin. Over the last seven years, at least one new research study investigating the effects of capsaicin has been published per day. Although researchers originally thought capsaicin worked primarily on nerves to reduce pain, recent studies have found that this amazing chemical is capable of much more.

Numerous studies have found that capsaicin profoundly influences many physiological processes: It reduces appetite; increases metabolism; lowers cholesterol; enhances the immune system; protects against cancer; makes insulin more effective; stops heart attacks; quiets an overactive bladder; prevents aspiration pneumonia (leading cause of death in the elderly); heals ulcers; clears up nasal congestion in allergies; reduces the size of nasal polyps; reduces pain in cluster headaches, diabetic neuropathy, postmastectomy pain syndrome, arthritis and atypical odontalgia (unusual pain condition with no effective treatment); reduces itching in psoriasis and in hemodialysis patients with uremia; counteracts the negative effects of stress; and may be beneficial in preventing Alzheimer's disease, Parkinson's disease and congestive heart failure, to name a few.

How Chilies Work

To understand how capsaicin works, it helps to have a grasp of how nerves function in the body. Nerves act as cables in the body, and transmit data such as pain, heat, touch and taste. This data is transmitted thorough the release of neurotransmitters (chemical messengers), such as serotonin, dopamine and acetylcholine.

When nerves feel a stimulus (pain, touch, taste or heat), it creates an electrical impulse. This electrical signal travels down the neuron (cables) until it reaches the end of the nerve (soma) and releases chemicals called neurotransmitters. The electrical charge signals the gatekeeper (ion channel) to open, which causes calcium to flow into the cell, and neurotransmitters to rush out. The released neurotransmitters then generate another electrical impulse to the adjacent nerve, which transmits the data. In short, pain, touch, heat or taste generates an electrical impulse, which then generates a chemical impulse (release of neurotransmitters), which acts to generate another electrical impulse to the next nerve. That's how nerves transmit data, or "talk to each other." Capsaicin works by changing how nerves talk to each other.

The short-term effect of capsaicin is that it makes nerves less excitable. The long-term effect is that it stops abnormal connections between neurons, which is called nerve plasticity. Two diseases that are linked to nerve plasticity are Alzheimer's and Parkinson's.

Interestingly, researchers have found that the brain cells that produce dopamine are destroyed in Parkinson's. Dopamine has also been linked to obesity. In a recent study, researchers found that severely obese people had fewer receptors for dopamine, and may need more food to feel full. Moreover, drugs used to treat schizophrenia that block dopamine make people put on weight, while drugs that boost dopamine levels (cocaine) reduce appetite and make people lose weight.

WHERE CAPSAICIN WORKS

Capsaicin affects many areas in the body, especially the cardiovascular, digestive and immune systems. The heart, digestive tract and respiratory tract are heavy innervated with nerves that are referred to as "capsaicin-sensitive" (nonmyelinated afferent fibers). These nerves respond more quickly to capsaicin because they lack (or have a thin covering of) a protective coating called myelin.

A key response of the body to capsaicin is vasodilation. Capsaicin causes blood vessels to dilate (open up), which increases blood flow, lowers blood pressure and promotes healing. Capsaicin also improves circulation by affecting the nerves that are responsible for directing blood flow to the heart, as well as the strength of the contractions of the blood vessels which push blood throughout the body.

Capsaicin stimulates nerves that activate the parasympathetic nervous system, which maintains many involuntary functions in the body—slowing the heart, increasing the activity in the gut, increasing salivation and constricting the bladder.

NEUROPEPTIDES

One of the most extensively studied effects of this fiery chemical is how it reduces pain. Capsaicin fights pain by entering the nerves and depleting them of substance P, a neuropeptide that transmits the pain signal to the brain. You release substance P when you burn your finger on the stove or stub your toe. Depleting the nerves of substance P stops pain signals in their tracks.

Capsaicin also alleviates pain by preventing the release of nerve growth factor (NGF), a substance that tells your nerves to make stronger connections between each other during the transmission of pain signals. A stronger connection between nerves is a situation you want to avoid when you hurt—it makes the pain more excruciating. Prenatally, NGF is needed for the development of the nervous system. After birth, a small population of cells lose their ability to respond to NGF, and begin to respond to glial cell line–derived neurotrophic factor (GDNF). Both NGF and GDNF have been shown to regulate the sensitivity of nerves that transmit pain signals (nociceptors) to both heat and capsaicin in adults.

Chilies and Children

Indigenous healers in Mexico and South America have an innate wisdom regarding this sacred plant—many advise nursing mothers to refrain from eating chilies (capsaicin may be transferred through breast milk) and to withhold foods that contain chilies from young children. This advice is prudent since their nervous system is still developing.

Chilies are introduced into a child's diet starting between the ages of four and six through chili-spiked salsas. The amount of chilies is gradually increased to acclimate a child's palate to this fiery fruit.

Another way chilies reduce pain is by releasing endorphins, your body's natural opiate. Opiates provide pain relief by stimulating gray neurons, which are attached to pain fibers. They reduce pain by clamping off the "cable" during the transmission of pain data between nerves. In a recent study, researchers found that a large dose of capsaicin produced the same degree of pain relief as 10 milligrams of morphine in rats.

However, that's only half the story. An element in your body called cholecystokinin, or CCK, lowers your sensitivity to morphine, and this is often high in diabetics who endure persistent, morphine-resistant pain. In a study conducted by Dr. Ghilardi et al., researchers found that capsaicin treatment down-regulated the production of CCK receptors, which resulted in a significant reduction of CCK binding sites. Perhaps capsaicin extinguishes pain not only by releasing endorphins, but also by making the body more sensitive to the opiates it secretes. This sacred plant appears to act in a synergistic way to make opiates more potent.

The beneficial effects of endorphins are not limited to pain relief. Endorphins also play a key role in decreasing the harmful effects of stress by reducing high levels of cortisol. This stress-based hormone not only increases your appetite for fats and carbs, but changes how and where your body stores fat.

STRESS FAT

Not all fat is created equal. While having thunder thighs may frustrate you, it doesn't pose the health risk of a large belly. In fact, the size of your belly is directly related to your risk of diabetes—your chances of developing diabetes are 40 percent if you have a large waist in contrast to only 6 percent if you have big hips!

Android obesity (central body fat) is defined by having a waist that measures thirty-five inches if you're a woman and forty inches for a man. Abdominal obesity is far more dangerous because this type of fat is more mobile. Central fat releases fatty acids into the liver, which controls a variety of metabolic functions in the body, including blood pressure, insulin and cholesterol levels.

Any fatty acid the liver doesn't use is returned to the central fat cells. As the central fat cells increase in size, they start dumping fatty acids into the bloodstream all the time, which causes insulin, cholesterol and blood pressure to shoot up. This increases your risk for heart disease, diabetes and cancer (breast, prostrate and colon). Pound for pound, researchers estimate that one pound of central body fat is approximately equivalent to eight pounds of lower body fat. Not a pretty picture.

Although you may not think so, you're lucky if have big thighs. Lower body fat, which is called gynecoid obesity, is found mostly below the skin (instead of near vital organs). This type of fat stays securely encased in fat cells and does not float around in the bloodstream.

While your genes are important for predicting where you wear your weight, stress also plays a very significant role. Stress can actually override genetics and shift your body from a lower body mode to a central body mode. Researchers have found that people with central fat tend to have more difficulty dealing with stress and are more likely to suffer from depression, have problems with alcohol or self-medicate with food.

It appears that the stress hormone, cortisol, is responsible for changing how and where you store your fat. Cortisol prompts glucose and fatty acids to be released, which provides energy to the muscles. However, the problem is that cortisol levels remain high even after the stress wanes. The result is that your body is taxed with a constant presence of fatty acids in the bloodstream, and your appetite increases to ensure that your body replaces the fuel it burned off.

The good news is that central fat is the first fat to be burned off when you work out. Exercise burns off the excess fatty acids that are released during stress so they no longer pose a risk to your health. Moreover, exercise prompts the brain to release endorphins, which calm us down and reduce cortisol levels.

It appears that managing stress is crucial to losing central fat. In a recent study conducted by Elissa Epel, diabetic men who used relaxation techniques to control stress lost a greater amount of central fat than the control group, which did not.

However, exercise isn't the only option for managing stress. Studies have shown that chilies, prayer and music also release endorphins, which facilitates a healthier lifestyle. Other options for reducing stress and cortisol levels include diaphragmatic breathing, meditation, massage, humor, aromatherapy and yoga.

Rate Your Risk

Central body fat is linked to heart disease, hypertension and diabetes because it causes a greater resistance to insulin, which contributes to these problems. Below are two ways to calculate if your belly puts you at risk:

1. Waist/Hip Ratio: calculate by dividing your waist measurement by your hip measurement.

Risk	Women	Men
Low risk	Less than 0.80	Less than 0.90
Moderate risk	0.80–0.85	0.90–1.0
High risk	Greater than 0.85	Greater than 1.02

2. Measure your waist: Women with a waist measurement over 35 inches are at risk; men with a waist measurement over 40 inches are at risk.

THE INSULIN CONNECTION

The body strives to maintain blood sugar levels (glucose) within a narrow range through the coordinated effort of several glands and their hormones. If these control mechanisms become disrupted, high blood sugar levels emerge.

The body responds to a rise in blood glucose after meals by releasing insulin, a hormone produced by the beta cells in the pancreas. Cells throughout your body (especially muscle cells) have receptors for insulin, which the insulin binds to after being released into your bloodstream. When insulin attaches to these receptors, a switch is activated, which starts a cascade of events that causes glucose to go to your cells and out of the bloodstream—that translates to a drop in blood sugar levels.

Insulin promotes the uptake of blood sugar by the cells of the body—it lowers blood glucose levels by increasing the rate at which cells throughout the body absorb glucose. However, when there is not enough insulin (type I diabetes), or when cells lack a sensitivity to it (type II), blood sugar cannot get into cells.

Up to 90 percent of all diabetics are type II diabetics. Typically, both insulin levels and blood sugar levels of these people are elevated, indicating that the insulin they're producing is no longer effective. In an effort to reduce high blood sugar levels, the pancreas continues to release larger amounts of insulin, but to no avail. Eventually, cells become so resistant to insulin that even enormous amounts won't move glucose into the cells.

Elevated levels of insulin wreck havoc in the body. They increase cholesterol levels and fat storage, and thicken arterial walls. Moreover, chronic high blood sugar levels, typically 140 mg/dl, damage many tissues, including the beta cells in the pancreas, which produce insulin. Eventually, the taxed cells in the pancreas stop producing insulin—a condition called "beta cell burnout." At this point, a type II diabetic converts to a type I diabetic and needs insulin replacement therapy.

The majority of individuals with type II diabetes are overweight. Achieving an ideal body weight restores normal blood sugar levels in many of these people. It appears that weight loss triggers the production of new, more efficient insulin receptors. However, some very intriguing animal studies have found that desensitizing certain capsaicin-sensitive nerves improves glucose tolerance. That means that less insulin was needed to lower high blood sugar levels.

Exactly how capsaicin achieves this remains unclear. For years, scientists have known that the sympathetic nervous system and the parasympathetic nervous system influence insulin secretion, and are involved in regulating blood sugar levels. However, the role of sensory nerves in maintaining blood sugar levels was a mystery. To unravel this riddle, scientists injected massive doses of capsaicin into newborn diabetic rats, which destroyed these nerves. This prevented the sensory nerves from releasing chemicals that are linked to increased insulin and blood sugar levels.

In an intriguing study conducted by Dr. Koopmans et al., researchers found that capsaicin increased the effectiveness of insulin in diabetic rats—by 21 percent! Capsaicin dramatically increased the capacity of muscles to pull glucose out of the bloodstream and store it as glycogen (a form of glucose that is stored in the muscles and liver), which lowered high blood sugar levels. Capsaicin achieved this by blocking the sensory nerves from releasing calcitonin gene-related peptide (CGRP), a neuropeptide which makes muscles less sensitive to insulin. And when muscles aren't sensitive to insulin, they remove less glucose from the blood. Moreover, capsaicin-treated diabetic rats had lower levels of certain hormones that fight the action of insulin and render it less effective.

EAT THE HEAT AND LOSE WEIGHT

Chilies help you lose weight in a variety of ways. First and fore-most, these pungent pods reduce your appetite, so that you eat less. Chilies make insulin more effective, which helps your body burn, rather than store, fat. Chilies release endorphins, so that you're less likely to binge under stress. These fiery fruits increase your metabolic rate, so that your body burns calories faster. Finally, chilies make low-fat food taste good, so that it's easier to stick to a diet.

Several studies have found that red pepper acts like a "non-pharmaceutical stimulant" and boosts the activity of the sympathetic nervous system. When this occurs you feel less hungry and eat less, although scientists can't pinpoint the exact reason why.

One theory for how chilies tame your appetite is that areas of the brain involved with satiety are richly innervated with nerves sensi-tive to capsaicin. Researchers have suggested that stimulating these nerves with capsaicin may trigger a response that reduces hunger.

Your gut has as many neurons as your brain, and it has been called the "second brain." The gut nervous system is very complex and has a dense network of both motor and sensory nerves. The motor nerves are responsible for moving food through your intestine, while the sensory nerves appear to influence appetite. Some researchers feel these nerves may be sensitive to capsaicin and send signals to the brain that you're "full" when exposed to this pungent chemical.

HOW CHILIES INCREASE METABOLISM

Studies have found that chilies increase the rate at which your body burns calories, a physiological process called thermogenesis. A chili-induced thermogenic burn helps you lose weight in two ways: It incinerates calories, and it prevents new fat from being formed.

Moreover, this calorie-blasting effect can last up to five hours after eating them.

In a study conducted at the Oxford Polytechnic Institute in England, researchers added a mixture of chili and hot mustard to the meals of twelve people, which increased metabolic rate by 25 percent—without exercise.

THE SCIENCE BEHIND THE CHILI PEPPER DIET

It's not news to anyone that to lose weight you need to eat less and exercise more. Although this prescription for weight loss sounds simple, it's not. One of the biggest stumbling blocks to weight loss is a feeling of being hungry: Most pharmaceutical weight-loss approaches have been directed at appetite suppression.

When you go on a low-fat diet, you force yourself to eat less. When you eat a chili-spiked diet, you *want* to eat less—that's the difference these fruits make! When chilies were added to meals in one study, people found that their hunger was markedly reduced. Not only did they eat less at that meal, they didn't feel hungry between meals. These pungent pods curbed appetite anywhere from two to four hours, which translated to eating less calories. And when that happened, people lost weight.

In the first part of the Chili Pepper Diet study (active period 1), chilies were added to several low-fat meals in fourteen people (ten women and four men). In the second part of the study (control period), chilies were removed from the low-fat diet. The third part of the study (active period 2), chilies were again added to the low-fat diet.

The results were amazing—a *tenfold* increase in weight loss occurred during the chili-spiked phase in contrast to the control period (no chilies). On average, people lost 9.4 pounds in an average of 56 days when they added chilies to their diet, but their weight loss plummeted to only 0.9 pounds during the phase with no chilies. When chilies were reintroduced into their diet, the pounds started to drop off again.

These results were accompanied by a highly significant p value of 0.0001. A p value is a number that denotes what the chances are that the study results occurred by random or chance. For instance, a p value of 0.05 means that there is a 5 percent chance the results occurred by coincidence, and a 95 percent chance that the results reflect what was manipulated in the study. Study results are considered significant (not by chance) if they are accompanied by a p value of 0.05. As the results of the Chili Pepper Diet emerged, it became clear that chilies were the missing link that made a low-fat diet work! This diet worked—and worked very well—in helping people lose weight!

A mantra for the Chili Pepper Diet emerged, "This does not *feel* like a diet." Within three weeks, the majority of the study participants stated they had lost their cravings for fatty foods and sweets. If they did eat these foods, it was at special occasions, and they were able to keep the portion sizes small. Cheating was no longer an issue since they no longer desired to eat these foods. What they *did* crave was chilies!

Other wonderful health benefits started to emerge—elevated blood sugar levels dropped and high blood pressure levels were reduced. Moreover, people reported getting a more restful night's sleep, their skin tones took on a rosy, healthy glow (capsaicin increases circulation), and they were better able to handle stress. One postmenopausal woman reported her sex drive increased!

GLUCOSE LEVELS

One participant was taking oral diabetic medication to control her high blood sugar, but it was not well controlled—her baseline glucose reading was 168. Within one month of eating a chili-spiked, low-fat diet, her blood sugar levels dropped to within normal limits—110. However, during the control period (no chilies) her blood sugar level jumped back to 160. After reintroducing chilies back into her low-fat diet, her blood sugar levels again started to decline.

Several other people who entered the diet study with elevated blood sugar levels also showed marked improvement. One person had an initial glucose level of 124. At the start of control, her glucose readings measured 114. By the end of the diet, her glucose was reading was a respectable 108. Another started the diet with a glucose reading of 187. After following the Chili Pepper Diet for several months, her glucose level dropped to 154. By the end of the diet, her glucose reading came in at 128. Although it's still higher than normal, it's a marked improvement. It's interesting that she did not eat chilies as frequently as the others. Also, the chilies she ate were mild (not as hot).

BLOOD PRESSURE

High blood pressure, or hypertension, is one of the most prevalent diseases in the United States. Approximately 50 million Americans over the age of sixty have high blood pressure, and 25 percent of American adults have high blood pressure. Hypertension contributes to heart disease and is closely linked to congestive heart failure and strokes.

Blood pressure is classified by different numbers. When you go to your doctor, the nurse will record two numbers when she takes your blood pressure—one number over another number. The top number is called the systolic number, and the bottom number is called the diastolic number. Normal blood pressure values occur when the top number is less than 130, and the bottom number is less than 85. Ideal blood pressure reading values are 120/80, or less. Hypertension is defined by readings of 140/90, or greater. Unfortunately, blood pressure tends to increase with age, especially systolic blood pressure.

Treating hypertension with medication isn't easy. Nearly half of patients give up on drugs because of side effects or expense. However, in ways that aren't fully understood, capsaicin lowers blood pressure by either causing blood vessels to relax, or by keeping them from constricting. In an intriguing animal study, researchers Nicholas Hadjokas and Theodore Goodfriend found that capsaicin reduces the production of a kidney hormone, aldosterone, that tightens blood vessels and causes the body to retain water. One of the most widely prescribed class drugs to treat mild to moderate hypertension, ACE inhibitors, also works by interfering with the production of this kidney hormone.

Lisa* (names have been changed to protect the privacy of the study participants) started the chili-enhanced diet with a blood pressure of 165/95. After eating a chili-enhanced diet for several months, her blood pressure dropped to 132/80. After maintaining a low-fat diet without chilies, her blood pressure had jumped back to 160/90 within four weeks. Yet, when chilies were added back into her diet, her blood pressure improved—it dropped to 130/80.

Another woman entered the study with a high blood pressure reading of 160/110. Within two weeks of eating chilies, her blood pressure dropped to 136/90.

CONTROLLING CRAVINGS

Many weight loss programs claim giving up sugar or fat prevents cravings. Yet, repeated studies have never confirmed that people really stop wanting fats and sweets. And there is a biochemical reason for this—stress depletes the brain of serotonin, a neurotransmitter that makes you feel calm, enhances your ability to concentrate and provides you with a deeper, more restful sleep. Stress also raises cortisol levels, which can trigger a binge.

When women feel stressed, they tend to reach for sweet/fatty foods, such as chocolate, ice cream and baked goods. Men often grab salty/fatty foods—steak, pizza and chips. Sound familiar? Yet, the common denominator in both of these food cravings is fat. Fats alleviate anxiety by triggering the body to release endorphins, which counteract the negative reaction of stress. However, using these foods as drugs has a price—your waistline. Chilies help control the cravings.

CHOCOLATE BINGES

The Mayas, Incas and Aztecs believed chocolate was a divine substance. And they might not have been too far from the truth. Chocolate is the most-craved food in this country—by a long shot. Nearly half of all food cravings are for chocolate. Many of us sip, bite and lick our way through twelve pounds of chocolate per year. Unfortunately, a 1.5-ounce chocolate bar also gives you half of your daily dose of saturated fat.

Chocolate cravings exist in 40 percent of women and 15 percent of men. There appears to be a strong hormonal link to chocolate cravings—they tend to be strongest just before and during a women's menstrual cycle. For one thing, estrogen levels take a dive just before women's periods. The problem is that when estrogen levels drop, so do levels of mood-boosting serotonin and endorphins, which makes most women feel irritable and more likely to binge on high-fat sweet foods.

This is also the time of the month when progesterone levels rise. In a study conducted by Buffensteine et al., researchers found that progesterone promotes fat storage, which may increase cravings for fatty foods.

However, that's only half the story. This "food of the gods" also contains chemicals that parallel those found in addictive substances. Small amounts of anadamine, a compound similar to the mood-altering chemicals in marijuana, is present in chocolate. Cocoa also contains phenylethylamine, a substance that's pharmacologically similar to amphetamines and increases your production of adrenaline and dopamine. However, it's chocolate's sensual texture and aroma that releases a flood of endorphins. Researchers postulate that people use chocolate as a drug to balance low levels of dopamine and endorphins, chemicals that are linked to overeating. Chilies have an amazing, not quite understood ability to halt these cravings in their tracks.

DIETING WITHOUT CHILIES

The amazing power of peppers to lower blood pressure, reduce hunger and cravings, facilitate weight loss, enhance mood and improve cholesterol profiles became even more apparent during the control period of the Chili Pepper Diet study. Within four days of eating a low-fat diet without chilies, cravings for fats and sweets emerged with a vengeance. Study participants stated that dieting had "become stressful or agonizing," and complained they felt "hungry," "lethargic," "angry," "anxious" and "deprived." Women upped their intake of starches, fats—*and chocolate*. Men cheated with fatty meats.

Moreover, maintaining reasonable portion sizes became a battle—a fight that many people lost.

These complaints were followed up with tangible results: People struggled to maintain their weight, slowed down their rate of weight loss or regained all the weight they had lost! In fact, one woman regained all the weight she had lost (twelve pounds) within four weeks.

Many of the study participants stated they just couldn't get a good night's sleep—either they were waking up too early, too often or their sleep just wasn't as restful. And less sleep makes weight loss harder—a lot harder. When you don't get enough sleep, cortisol levels increase. This stress-based hormone not only ups insulin levels, but also increases the activity of a lipoprotein lipase, an enzyme that prompts the body to store fat.

CHOLESTEROL LEVELS

Coronary artery disease (CAD) is the leading cause of death in both men and women. Over 10 million Americans suffer from coronary artery disease, and many more are undiagnosed. More than five hundred thousand people a year die from heart disease, and the resulting medical costs are in the range of 50 to 100 billion dollars a year—a staggering number!

Coronary artery disease occurs when fatty deposits (plaque) develop in the inside of the arteries and clog them. These plaques, which develop over time, are made of cholesterol and other substances that slowly go bad. As a plaque develops in an artery, the artery begins to narrow and restricts the ability of blood to flow to the heart or the brain, which leads to a heart attack or stroke.

While a diet high in saturated fats will raise cholesterol levels in many people, others naturally produce too much cholesterol. Both situations contribute to a poor cholesterol profile and increase your risk for heart disease.

The American Heart Association and National Cholesterol Education Program advocate that you reduce fat calories and replace them with carbohydrate calories to lower cholesterol levels. However, heart-protective HDL levels fall and triglyceride levels rise if you don't lose weight, or get lots of exercise. Unfortunately, most Americans can't stick to a low-fat diet and regain the weight they lost. And there's a reason why this occurs. In a study published in the *International Journal of Obesity and Related Metabolic Disorders*, researchers found that losing weight on a low-fat diet and exercise regimen increased cortisol levels, and upped people's appetite. Moreover, this type of diet jacked up hunger levels to a greater extent in men.

Adding chilies to your diet will improve your body's ability to process both cholesterol and fats. Capsaicin accomplishes this in two ways: It decreases the absorption of cholesterol and increases enzymes in the liver that are responsible for fat metabolism. This prompts the liver to secrete, rather than store, triglycerides. In a study published in *Atherosclerosis*, researchers found that a component of capsaicin, dihydrocapsaicin, lowers LDL and increases HDL cholesterol.

In the Chili Pepper Diet, high cholesterol levels showed a dramatic improvement. LDL cholesterol (the bad kind) was reduced by 21 percent, total cholesterol was lowered by 12 percent, while HDL cholesterol (the good kind) and triglyceride levels stayed close to baseline levels.

Results of the Chili Pepper Diet on Cholesterol Levels

	Baseline	End of Diet	P value
LDL	134.45 mg/dl	106.049 mg/dl	0.0003
TC	210.50 mg/dl	184.560 mg/dl	0.015
TG	140.11 mg/dl	140.167 mg/dl	not significant
HDL	52.90 mg/dl	51.65 mg/dl	not significant

In the first few weeks of the diet, there was a decline in both LDL cholesterol and HDL cholesterol. However, HDL levels jumped back up within three weeks in some, while it took several months in others. Some people increased their HDL levels when they reached their goal weight—at that point it shot up.

While triglycerides increased at the beginning of the study, this was only temporary. Triglycerides levels naturally increase during weight loss. However, elevated triglyceride levels become a concern if they remain elevated after you lose weight. As people lost weight, reached their goal weight or their body adjusted to the diet, triglyceride levels fell back to baseline, or below baseline, levels.

It was intriguing that HDL levels exceeded (increased by 14 points) baseline levels in several patients who reached their goal weight. This is unusual since weight loss partially offsets drops in HDL levels on low-fat diets. While losing weight will prompt HDL levels to climb back up, they often don't reach baseline levels.

Many weight-loss programs advocate walking for at least thirty minutes per day, while extremely low-fat diets require much more. Exercise is crucial in a low-fat diet—it offsets drops in HDL cholesterol and lowers high triglycerides. And the lower the fat content, the more you need to work out. Very low-fat diets advocate one hour of exercise—a level which most Americans can't maintain.

In the Chili Pepper Diet, most people followed a realistic exercise regime: walking at a brisk pace for thirty minutes at the rate of three to four times per week. Lori joined the program because she wanted to lose twenty pounds. She entered the program with a good cholesterol profile: total cholesterol was 160 mg/dl, HDL was measured at 49 mg/dl, LDL cholesterol was 92 mg/dl and triglycerides were 95 mg/dl. After losing twenty-two pounds, her total cholesterol dropped to an impressive 149 mg/dl, HDL increased to 56 mg/dl, LDL was lowered to 75 mg/dl and triglycerides fell to 89 mg/dl. Considering her exercise regime was moderate (she walked for thirty minutes three to four times per week), these results were impressive! It appears that chilies augmented the beneficial effects of exercise!

Alan's goal was to lose only ten pounds—that's it. His cholesterol wasn't a concern: TC was 117 mg/dl, HDL was 38 mg/dl, LDL came in at 70 mg/dl and triglycerides were 44 mg/dl. After losing close to eight pounds, his cholesterol numbers were remarkable considering he did a minimal amount of exercise: His HDL (the good kind) increased to 52 mg/dl (fourteen-point increase). Larry entered the program with a low HDL level of 29 mg/dl. However, after being on the program for three months, his HDL increased to 42 mg/dl. His exercise was moderate—he walked for thirty minutes per day at the rate of three times per week.

The ability of chilies to lower LDL (the bad kind) cholesterol levels and maintain HDL (the good kind) cholesterol levels became even more apparent during the period when chilies were withheld in the diet (control period). This was most pronounced in people who ate more chilies than others. Mary ate several chilies with each meal—including snacks. Her HDL levels had increased from a baseline reading of 47 mg/dl to 53 mg/dl during four weeks of the diet. However, during control (no chilies), her HDL dropped to

34 mg/dl. After adding chilies back into her diet, her HDL jumped to 51 mg/dl in two months.

This seems to support what numerous studies have found—weight loss and exercise are not the definitive answer to the problems of a low-fat diet. However, when you factor chilies into the equation—it works.

DEPRESSION

A situation occurred during the control period (no chilies) of the study that was not anticipated. Two women who had a prior history of depression complained they started feeling depressed. They felt "sad," "moody," "tired" and "irritable." One woman stated she had trouble managing her anger—everyday annoyances now escalated to family fights. By the third week of the control period, she stated dieting had become "difficult" and requested, "to be put back on chilies, or be given a prescription for Prozac." The first morning after control, she celebrated by eating six jalapenos at breakfast. Within four days of going back on chilies, she stated she felt more relaxed, her complexion was glowing, she was getting a better night's sleep and her hunger was, once again, under control.

HOW CHILIES DECREASE
YOUR RISK FOR HEART DISEASE

The risk of heart disease can be reduced by 60 percent by making certain lifestyle changes—reducing high cholesterol levels, losing weight, lowering high blood pressure, exercising and not smoking. In many cases, high cholesterol levels can be reduced by making changes in your diet, which involves *restricting* certain foods in your diet, while *adding* others. The good news is that adding chilies to your diet can reduce many of these risks.

It's crucial to reduce the amount of saturated fats you eat, which the liver uses to manufacture cholesterol. Saturated fats are found in animal products (dairy products and fatty meats) and some vegetable products (coconut oil, palm oil and hydrogenated oils). Also, you should avoid products that use partially hydrogenated fats, which many researchers feel are just as bad as, if not worse than, saturated fats.

However, you also need to add heart-healthy foods to your diet. Eat more fatty fish rather than chicken or beef. Replace refined carbohydrates with complex carbohydrates, such as whole grains, beans, fresh fruits and vegetables. Add chilies to your menu plan and eat them throughout the day. Use monounsaturated fats to flavor, rather than fry, your food. These changes in your diet will help you lose weight. They will also provide protection against heart disease by keeping your LDL cholesterol low and your HDL cholesterol high. Moreover, these dietary changes will lower your triglycerides and reduce your blood pressure. If you pair these dietary changes with moderate amounts of exercise, you'll see results!

THE FIVE CONTROLLABLE RISK FACTORS FOR HEART DISEASE

There are certain risk factors that you can't change, such as your age, family history and gender. That's the hand nature dealt you. However, you can control five risk factors: high cholesterol levels, high blood pressure, being overweight, smoking and exercise. The good news is that adding chilies to your diet can significantly reduce many of these risks.

In men, being older than forty-five years of age is a risk factor. In women, being older than fifty-five years old is considered a risk factor. A ten-year lag is seen in women because female hormones give them a protective edge. However, by age fifty-five, women no longer have the protective effect female hormones provide, and they have the same potential for developing heart disease as men.

Family history is definitely a risk factor. Unfortunately, it is one you can't change. Family history is defined as having a first-degree relative (mother, father, sister or brother) who had a heart attack before the age of fifty-five, which puts you at a higher risk of having a heart attack yourself.

Another risk factor you can't change is being menopausal. It is believed that the female hormone, estrogen, protects a woman against heart disease by changing her cholesterol profile. When estrogen levels drop, LDL cholesterol (the bad kind) increases, HDL cholesterol (the good kind) decreases and the total cholesterol increases as well. These negative changes contribute to the development of heart disease.

Women younger than forty-five usually have a total cholesterol that ranges from 185 to 207. However, women older than forty-five typically range from 217 to 237, while 50 percent of women over the age of fifty-five top 240. A desirable total cholesterol reading is below 200. A borderline high reading is considered 200 to 239, while 240 is considered high.

There are marked differences in risk factors between the sexes for cardiovascular disease as well. For instance, diabetes is a much stronger risk for women. Moreover, there is a greater chance you will die from cardiovascular disease if you have diabetes. In fact, the negative health effects of diabetes are so strong that they actually negate the protection most women receive from estrogen.

Two very important cholesterol numbers are your HDL and triglycerides, especially in women. The higher a HDL cholesterol number is, the more protected you are. A high HDL cholesterol level will offer protection against heart disease in spite of high LDL cholesterol. Moreover, a high HDL cholesterol level (the good kind) has a stronger protective effect in women. For instance, an HDL cholesterol level of 45, rather than 35, is considered low.

A high triglyceride level is not a number you want to see—levels over 200 milligrams are now considered an independent risk factor for heart disease. Also, triglyceride levels over 200 are a stronger predictor for heart disease in women than men.

People who don't exercise have a more difficult time managing their weight and tend to have higher cholesterol numbers. Exercise becomes extremely important as we age—it conditions the heart and decreases our chances of becoming overweight.

Weigh Your Risk

As your Body Mass Index (BMI) tops 25, your risk for heart disease goes up dramatically.

Height	25 BMI "overweight"	30 BMI "obese"
4'10"	119 lbs.	143 lbs.
4'11"	124 lbs.	148 lbs.
5'	128 lbs.	153 lbs.
5'1"	132 lbs.	158 lbs.
5'2"	136 lbs.	164 lbs.
5'3"	141 lbs.	169 lbs.
5'4"	145 lbs.	174 lbs.
5'5"	150 lbs.	180 lbs.
5'6"	155 lbs.	186 lbs.
5'7"	159 lbs.	191 lbs.
5'8"	164 lbs.	197 lbs.
5'9"	169 lbs.	203 lbs.
5'10"	174 lbs.	207 lbs.
5'11"	179 lbs.	215 lbs.
6'	184 lbs.	221 lbs.

Eating chilies can reduce many of the risk factors that contribute to heart disease: They will lower high cholesterol, reduce high blood sugar, help you lose weight, decrease high blood pressure and alleviate stress. Moreover, some intriguing research has found that capsaicin may help prevent congestive heart failure, a condition that is characterized by an enlarged heart.

It's astounding that a fruit is capable of doing so much good. And it costs only pennies a day for this truly miraculous food. I can only imagine what a pharmaceutical company would charge for a such a drug.

BOOSTING THE EFFECTS OF EXERCISE

Starting at age twenty-five, a woman starts to lose a half pound of muscle tissue per decade—that translates to a 5 percent decrease in her metabolic rate. If 2,000 calories per day maintained her weight at age twenty, that number will drop to 1,800 calories per day by the time she hits forty. And if she continues to eat the same amount of calories as the years go by without upping her exercise, she will gain around one pound per year after thirty-five. Although men also have to contend with muscle loss and fat gain in mid-life, women lose twice as much muscle and gain twice as much fat.

You can turn the tide with exercise and chilies. Exercise tames your appetite by releasing dopamine, serotonin, noradrenaline and adrenaline. Exercise also increases muscle tissue, which burns fat. Moreover, exercise increases your body's ability to use oxygen (oxygen consumption rate), which is a key factor in burning fat.

Exercised muscles have a greater ability to pull fat and glucose from the blood. If you exercise for several months, you can increase your oxygen consumption rate by approximately 15 percent. This calorie-blasting effect can last anywhere from one to five hours after

A Low-Fat Diet with and Without Chilies
Adjusted LDL Means

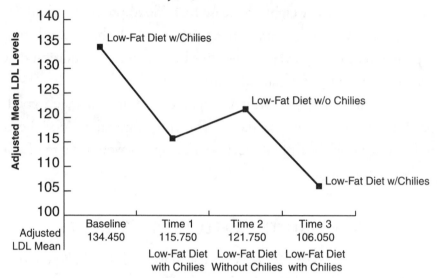

Adjusted LDL Mean	Baseline 134.450	Time 1 115.750	Time 2 121.750	Time 3 106.050
		Low-Fat Diet with Chilies	Low-Fat Diet Without Chilies	Low-Fat Diet with Chilies

A Low-Fat Diet with and Without Chilies
Mean Weight (Arithmetic)

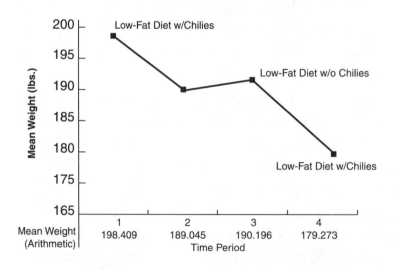

Mean Weight (Arithmetic)	1 198.409	2 189.045	3 190.196	4 179.273

Time Period

Control Period 1: A low-fat, high-fiber diet with chilies: People experienced reduced appetite and cravings, stayed on the diet and consistently lost weight.

Control Period 2: A low-fat, high-fiber diet without chilies: Appetite increased and rate of weight loss slows; many people regained lost weight.

Control Period 3: Back on a low-fat, high-fiber diet with chilies: People's appetite is reduced and they stayed on the diet. They progressively lost weight.

you work out. And it's not just the number of calories that are burned during your workout, but the increased rate that calories are burned after exertion which helps you lose weight.

Studies have shown that eating chilies can mirror the beneficial effects of exercise in several ways: They increase your metabolic rate, up the rate at which your body uses oxygen and counteract stress by releasing endorphins. In a Korean study, researchers L. Kiwon et al. found that chilies both increased oxygen consumption rate (13 percent) and metabolic rate (10 percent) in endurance athletes—*at rest!* To put this in perspective, exercising for at least thirty minutes boosts your metabolism 10 percent for one hour after you've worked out.

So, as you can see from the research, adding chilies to your diet will help you lose weight faster and keep it off. Moreover, these pungent pods will improve your capacity to process fats, cholesterol and sugar, which translates to reducing your risk for heart disease, diabetes and strokes. So, spice up your meals and jump-start your way to a slimmer you and better health.

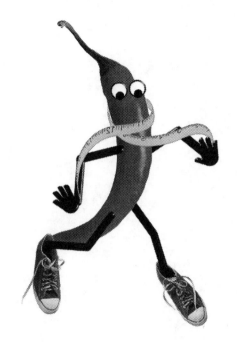

Part II

THE
CHILI PEPPER
DIET

CHAPTER THREE

USE FLAVOR—NOT FAT

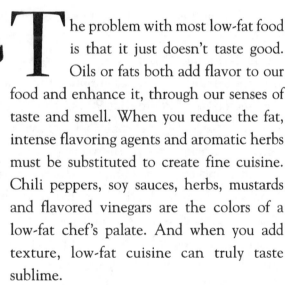

The problem with most low-fat food is that it just doesn't taste good. Oils or fats both add flavor to our food and enhance it, through our senses of taste and smell. When you reduce the fat, intense flavoring agents and aromatic herbs must be substituted to create fine cuisine. Chili peppers, soy sauces, herbs, mustards and flavored vinegars are the colors of a low-fat chef's palate. And when you add texture, low-fat cuisine can truly taste sublime.

To create flavor, you must first understand the biologic functions involved in the perception of taste, the connection between aroma and taste which defines flavor and the principles of combining flavors. Working with taste-enhancing agents requires knowledge and practice, but you'll soon see the reward. Well-prepared low-fat cuisine satisfies both your body and your soul—it not only tastes good, it makes you feel good.

THE TASTE-AROMA CONNECTION

The word "flavor" is derived from the Old French word *flaor*, meaning "aroma." Even back then, the French understood that the sense of smell was connected to the sense of taste and used aroma to make their food more enticing. Our sense of smell is so intertwined with our sense of taste that aroma can actually define flavor. To prove this point, do a simple experiment. Put a piece of pear under your nose and bite into an apple. What you'll taste is a pear. And did you know that vanilla is not a taste but a scent? Bakeries use vanilla for its sweet perfume, not its bitter taste, to enhance the flavor of desserts.

Researchers estimate that 90 percent of a food's taste comes from its smell. Recently, neurobiologists have confirmed the odor/taste connection originates in the most primitive areas of the brain, the amygdala and the hippocampus, which are part of the limbic system. Aroma activates taste, which are paired in the brain to create flavor. This process begins when odor molecules sniffed by the nose are picked up by the cilia, hairlike projections in the olfactory nerve cells, and are translated by electrical signals to the limbic system (part of the brain responsible for emotions). There the brain stores the scent in its memory banks where the association of what you smelled with what you tasted is filed.

Only four elementary tastes are actually perceived by the tongue: salty, sour, bitter and sweet. All subtle flavors, like vanilla, are actually aromas. And sensory cells in the nose are much more discerning than your tongue. That is why people who have lost their sense of smell, because of colds, flu or chronic sinus problem, usually can't taste their food.

However, researchers are currently looking into the possibility of a fifth perceivable flavor—meat. The Japanese call it *umami*, and with 20 percent of the population craving this flavor, the addition of meat-flavored chilies is indispensable to making a low-fat diet palatable!

To make truly delicious low-fat cuisine, you need to incorporate aroma to enhance its flavor. Using aromatic herbs such as rosemary, garlic, mesquite and smoked chilies will go a long way to making your food taste better. Aroma is the talisman for creating great-tasting low-fat cuisine.

Aroma can also help you lose weight. Your desire to eat is greatly influenced by the limbic system, which can be tamed by smell. This is part of the magic of the Chili Pepper Diet!

THE SCIENCE OF FLAVOR COMBINATIONS

Researchers used to think only the tongue perceived taste—identifying salty, sweet, sour and bitter flavors. However, recent studies have found taste buds are actually housed throughout the oral cavity—on the tongue, palate, epiglottis, larynx and esophagus. There is a close relationship between pain and taste because the nerves that sense temperature and pain are wrapped around the taste receptors. For instance, the pain receptors that sense high temperatures also are activated by the chemical in chilies, capsaicin. That's why spicy food tastes "hot" even if it's cold. Flavor is really aroma plus taste plus pain.

Chemicals occurring naturally in foods can be used to heighten flavor. The chemical found in chilies, capsaicin, is the most aggressive of these. Capsaicin is eight times more pungent than the chemical found in black pepper, peperine. Gingerols, the compounds found in ginger, are more subtle. Chilies, onions, horseradish, mustards and radishes—which all contain taste-enhancing chemicals—are necessary ingredients in any low-fat program. They make the food seem more flavorful by activating both the pain receptors and the taste buds. In low-fat cuisine, "two is better than one."

Flavors can be broken down into two categories: primary and secondary. Primary flavors are the most pronounced; they seem to jump off the plate and onto your tongue. The rosemary in rosemary chicken is a good example of a primary flavor. In chicken marsala, the marsala is the dominant taste; and in hollandaise sauce, it's the lemon that catches your attention.

Secondary flavors, which are more subtle than primary flavor, add "depth" to a dish. That is, they enhance the primary flavor by making it more complex. For instance, carrots taste even sweeter with a little grated ginger; a squeeze of lime juice in black bean chili adds zest without leaving a citrus tone; and butternut squash soup comes alive with a splash of brandy. It can be difficult to pinpoint these ingredients, but there's no doubt that foods just taste better with them. They are those "secret" ingredients that add magic to a dish.

Flavor Marriage

If you could compare flavor to music, flavor marriage would be jazz. It's mellow and soothing. Combining primary and secondary flavors creates dishes that have complexity and depth. When you blend flavors it's crucial to know which flavors enhance rather than repel one another to create a balanced presentation.

Some flavors "marry" to form a single taste. For instance, in Creole cuisine, onion, celery and bell peppers are blended to form one taste, called the Holy Trinity. It is the base of many uptown New Orleans dishes. Indian curry and Mexican mole work in much the same way:

combinations of three to twelve spices are blended to form one recognizable taste. You master flavor marriage through experience because some combinations work and some don't. It takes practice!

Some flavors that marry well in low-fat cuisine include caramelized onions, celery and bell peppers; rice wine vinegar and tarragon; molasses and ginger; lemon and caramelized garlic; thyme and mushrooms; tarragon and apples; and shellfish and curry powder.

Flavor Opposition

Flavor opposition creates bold, exciting cuisine. Like rock-and-roll music, it energizes you. Flavors that oppose each other—sweet/hot, sweet/salty, sweet/sour, salty/tart and salty/hot—either heighten or cancel each other out depending on the proportions used. Flavor opposition is easier to achieve than flavor marriage because it follows this cardinal rule: Add a little of the first ingredient to the second ingredient. For instance, frosting is a sweet/salty combination. If you add a little salt to the sugar mixture, it tastes sweeter. If you add equal amounts of sugar and salt, you get a neutral taste that is neither sweet nor salty.

Asian chefs, in particular, have elevated using flavor opposition to an art form. For example, to counter the salty taste of their soy sauce, Japanese chefs add mirin, a sweet rice wine, or, alternatively, citrus juice. Thai chefs add chilies to nampla to temper the salt and heighten the flavor of this fish-based soy sauce. Opposing flavors that work well in low-fat cuisine include: Dijon mustard and peppers; fruit and chili powder; rice wine vinegar and chili; soy sauce and chili; soy sauce and mirin; and smoked chilies and ketchup.

TEXTURE

Fats not only flavor food, they also provide texture. Fats and oils make a cake moist, a sauce rich and creamy and give Southern fried chicken its crunch. Creating texture is the most challenging task in creating low-fat cuisine. It requires combining cooking techniques with a variety of nonfat products to mimic the functions of oil. But take heart, it can be done!

And while vegetables and grains create texture, they do so only if they are fresh. Take the time to select vegetables that feel firm to the touch and have vibrant color.

Sauces: Cooking Them the Chili Pepper Way

Cream sauces. To create a rich, thick nonfat cream sauce, combine canned skim milk and defatted chicken stock and use a cooking technique called reduction (which produces a thick texture). In reduction, you boil off the excess liquid through evaporation. However, the trick is to use a high heat and shake your nonstick pan back and forth continuously while reducing the liquid. As the excess liquid boils off through evaporation, the protein molecules roll over each other, which thickens the sauce to the consistency of a full-fat cream. (Once you start shaking the pan, don't stop or the sauce will be thin and runny.)

Vegetable-based cream sauce. Pureed parsnips taste more like cream than other vegetables (such as potatoes). You'll save 44 grams of fat substituting parsnips for half a cup of cream in soups or sauces.

Broth-based sauces or soups. Pureed starches or legumes thicken broth-based soups or sauces. For instance, if you add a few tablespoons of steamed rice or a corn tortilla to a thin soup, it will give it "body." First, combine your ingredients in a blender (for 5 to 6 seconds), then transfer them to a pan and reheat. This "trick" will give you the same results as cream or butter.

Baked goods. Add pureed bananas, prunes, raisins and applesauce to baked goods to keep them soft and moist. This technique will replace up to seven-eighths of the butter or shortening called for in traditional recipes and is more nutritious because fruits provide fiber, antioxidants and phytochemicals. You will get the best results if the fruit is pureed to the consistency of butter; the most convenient form is unsweetened baby food.

1. Fresh fruit purees, such as mashed bananas and applesauce, work best in muffins, pancakes and light cakes.
2. Raisin pastes are the best choice for dense, chewy cookies.
3. Pureed prunes are the best substitutes for butter in chocolate-flavored desserts.

Sautéing

Substituting wine and stock for oils while sautéing will omit 14 grams of fat per serving. However, your success will depend upon two factors—choosing the correct stand-in for each dish and using the right amounts. In general, replacing 4 tablespoons of wine or stock per 1 tablespoon of oil in a recipe will produce the best results.

Red wines. Use in tomato-based dishes. You will get the best flavor if you sauté the onions and garlic in wine for pasta sauces.

Fruity wines. Use a medium-dry white wine (sauvignon blanc) instead of olive oil when preparing seafood. Do not use a dry white wine—it leaves a metallic taste. Use a fruity or blush wine for fruit-based desserts.

Veal stock. Use in dishes that call for lean pork, mushrooms, pasta, root vegetables or veal—it enhances "earthy" flavors and creates a rich taste. My favorite stock!

Chicken. A good, all-purpose stand-in for any dish calling for olive oil. Adds a richer flavor than vegetable stocks.

Vegetable. A good choice in vegetarian-style meals.

Nonfat "Frying"

Producing a crust without oil is the most difficult task in low-fat cooking. However, you can "fry" foods using several techniques.

Baking. Cover bread-crumb-coated foods with a nonstick spray before baking.

Grilling. When you use a grill or broiler, the high temperature caramelizes animal proteins such as fish or poultry, which naturally produces a crustlike "skin."

Pan frying. Using a little kosher salt in a heavy-weight stainless steel pan will duplicate pan frying without the use of oil. The food gets a crust without sticking to the pan. This technique works especially well with ground turkey and chicken.

Putting It All Together

Now that we've covered the principles involved, let's take a look at the specific flavor-enhancing agents and techniques for preparation that you'll use in the recipes of this book in Part Three.

Low-Fat Flavoring Agents

Sauces

Dark soy sauce. A Chinese soy sauce that is made from fermented soybeans and water. Has both a sweet and salty taste.

Mirin. Syrupy wine made from short-grained glutenous rice and 90-proof Shochu liquor. Adds sheen and sweetness to food.

Mushroom-flavored soy sauce. A thick, dark soy sauce that tastes like a concentrated mushroom stock.

Nampala. A thin, amber-colored Thai soy sauce made from anchovies or shrimp. It adds depth to a dish without lending a fishy taste when used in small amounts. Much lower in sodium than regular soy sauce. A "secret" ingredient in most Thai food.

Ponzu sauce. A thin Japanese soy sauce that is made from fermented soybeans, water and citrus juice. This works wonders on grilled fish and steamed veggies.

Sake. A Japanese wine brewed from steamed rice and purified water. The amino acids (proteins) in the wine tenderize foods and balance the flavor of the salt in the soy sauce.

Vinegars

Balsamic. An Italian vinegar that is mild and sweet. Is aged in oak casks like a fine cognac and its cost ranges from $5.00 to $150.00 for an 8-ounce bottle. (It's worth it to spend at least $10.00 a bottle to get a superior product that does not taste acidic.) A fine balsamic is concentrated flavor that you use drop by drop. It enhances the flavor of spicy salad greens such as watercress and arugula and also the bitter lettuces: radicchio, Belgian endive and chicory. Add a spicy Dijon mustard, tarragon, chilies, shallots and half a teaspoon of olive oil for a delicious low-fat vinaigrette.

Chili. Has a spicy/tart or spicy/sweet taste, depending on the ingredients used. Since there are few commercial products on the market, I create my own by heating various vinegars and chili. Enhances the flavor of poultry, salads, fish, seafood, meat, vegetables, grains and legumes.

Cider. Has a tart, citrus flavor and the aroma of apples, from which it is derived. Its fruity flavor sweetens when heated and combines well with smoked chicken and turkey.

Distilled white. Tastes less acidic compared to plain white vinegar and is a good choice for pickling cucumbers and chilies. Enhances the flavor of bean dips, salad dressings and salsas.

Fruit-flavored. Prepared from fruits and white wine, these vinegars add both a fruity aroma and flavor. They enhance the flavor of fruit and poultry salads. Pineapple vinegar is the best choice for pickling chilies.

Herb. Made from herbs, such as tarragon, added to white wine vinegar. Best used with bitter lettuces such as Belgian endive, radicchio and chicory, or milder-tasting ones such as butter, red leaf or romaine. Clashes with the "spicy" lettuces: arugula and watercress.

Rice wine. A Japanese vinegar that is mild and sweet. I prefer the seasoned rice wine vinegar over the regular rice wine vinegar because it's less acidic and has mellower taste, the greatest gift to low-fat cuisine since nonfat yogurt! Wonderful on salads with a little dried tarragon.

Citrus Juices

Lemon. As opposed to the distinctiveness of lime, this flavor blends into a dish. Useful for cleaning foods, such as chicken and fish, before cooking or adding "sparkle" to green vegetables.

Lime. The most versatile citrus juice, it is used for its distinctive flavor and acidity. Lime enhances the sweetness of fruit and heightens the flavor of salsas and Caribbean black bean soups. Pick large, yellow limes, which have a better flavor and more juice.

Orange. Blends well with carrots and the sweet squashes, such as butternut.

Mustards

Dijon. A French white wine mustard with a spicy hot flavor that marries beautifully with smoked poultry. The flavor is enhanced with pickled peppers and works well in a balsamic vinaigrette.

Dijon with horseradish. Has a thicker texture, tastes less acidic and is not as spicy compared to regular Dijon. Enhances the flavor of smoked poultry and root vegetables.

German. A grainy brown mustard that has a sweet, hearty flavor without the bite of a French Dijon. The flavor is enhanced with sweet chilies.

Honey mustard. Has a thin, creamy texture and a sweet taste. Works well as part of a marinade for poultry, in salad dressings or as a glaze over carrots.

Salts

Iodized. I never use this product because it has no flavor.

Kosher. Professional chefs use kosher salt as a flavoring catalyst—it brightens the flavor of foods. You'll use less salt (merely $\frac{1}{16}$ of a teaspoon) to flavor food with this product because you don't measure it with a spoon—simply grab a little between your thumb and index and middle fingers and grind it over the food. Keep a dish of this salt on your stove and use at the sauté stage for caramelizing vegetables (onions and garlic) and sprinkle on fish, chicken or meat at the end of food preparation.

Sea. Has good flavor but, unlike kosher salt, is inconvenient to use because you have to grind it. It's also more expensive than kosher salt.

Spices and Herbs

Achiote paste. An aromatic Mexican (Yucatan region) seasoning paste made from ground annatto seeds, cumin, cinnamon, cloves and oregano. Should be cooked before use to remove chalky taste. Thinned with citrus juices and used in a marinade for grilled poultry, it adds a subtle sweet flavor and a beautiful yellow hue to food.

Cardamom. Lends a sweet, slightly lemony flavor that enhances the taste of sweet vegetables and fruits. Especially good with melons, carrots, rice and sweet potatoes.

Chilies. Chilies not only provide heat but also flavor. These fruits can taste like nuts, chocolate, fruits or meat. Chilies are indispensable to a low-fat diet; they liven the taste of grains, legumes, vegetables, fruit, fish, chicken and meat, and, of course, you can't follow the Chili Pepper Diet without them. Dried chilies can be ordered online at *www.monterreyfoodsproducts.com* and *www.chiliguy.com*.

Cilantro (Chinese parsley or fresh coriander). Used in Oriental, North African, Indian, Indonesian and Mexican cuisine, this zesty herb lends a warm-bodied taste to highly seasoned dishes. Use only the leaves and tender stems (tough stems can taste bitter). Store this herb in the refrigerator with the root ends in a glass of water and the leaves covered with a plastic bag for up to two weeks to preserve its freshness. So unique, cilantro cannot be substituted.

Cumin. An Egyptian herb indispensable to Mexican, North African, Middle Eastern, Thai, Indian and Southwestern American cuisine. The rich flavor of the flat, brown oval seeds is enhanced by pan-toasting before use (heat releases the oils which contain the flavor). Once the seed is crushed, it has a short shelf life. Available at Indian and Mexican markets. Enhances the flavor of cabbage, rice, sauces and dishes that contain chilies.

Curry powder. Curry is a blend of seeds (cumin, black mustard, coriander, fenugreek), spices (chilies, peppercorns, turmeric) and ground curry leaves. It enhances stewed vegetables (carrots, cauliflower, onions, potatoes and tomatoes), seafood, fish and poultry. Cook briefly in a small amount of oil to release flavor. The best commercial curry is obtained in Indian markets.

Garam masala. Originating in the colder climates of North India, people use this spice to generate internal body heat. Garam masala is a blend of dry-roasted "warm" spices—black pepper, cardamom, chilies, cinnamon, cloves, coriander, cumin, ginger and mace—which "marry" to form a single taste. Masala can be used as either "dry seasonings" or as "wet seasonings" (a combination of dry spices and liquids). However, dry masalas should be used at the end of the cooking process or as a garnish, like paprika. The best masala is homemade, which you create by grinding together four to six spices with a mortar and pestle. If you don't have the time to make your own, buy a product that is sold in resealable vacuum-packed tins (flavor is preserved better than if stored in a cellophane package). This can be obtained in Indian markets or in the ethnic section of the supermarkets. Enhances the flavor of vegetables, grains, legumes, poultry, fish and meats.

Ginger. This root is relished for its medicinal properties and invigorating sharp, sweet taste. Buy fresh ginger that is firm to the touch with a smooth, unwrinkled skin. Ginger enhances the taste of apples, melons, carrots, onions, sweet potatoes, squashes, fish, red lentils, chicken and beef.

Horseradish. This pungent root contains a phytochemical, isocanthates, which has both medicinal and culinary properties. However, it must be used within a few hours after grating or its pungency fades. Use fresh (not dried) for the best flavor, and avoid the skin and woody inner core. It enhances the flavor of root vegetables such as potatoes or yams.

Mexican oregano. This spice has a sweeter, more delicate flavor than Greek oregano and it works better in dishes that contain chilies. Toast in a pan if using the dried form to bring out its full flavor. Mexican oregano can be obtained through mail-order catalogues, online at *www.monterreyfoodsproducts.com* or in Latin markets.

Mustard seeds (black). Used in Indian cooking, these seeds lend a nutty flavor to foods. Before use, pan-toast the seeds till they "pop" to release their flavor. They enhance the taste of curries, sauces and salads.

Rosemary. This aromatic herb should be used in its dried form; fresh rosemary tastes like pine tar and has a woody texture. It enhances the flavor of breads, stuffing, soups and poultry.

Seasoning pastes. In Mexico, most markets sell these seasoning pastes—recado, adobodo, chilaqil, salpimentado and alcaparrdo—already made up in the correct proportions. Recado, a mixture of garlic, dried chilies and spices, is used as a dry spice rub before grilling. Adobodo, consisting of dried chilies and sometimes vinegar, is used to marinate meat, fish and poultry before grilling or roasting.

Sumac (dried pomegranate). Used in Indian and Iranian food, dried ground pomegranate imparts a sweet-and-sour taste. It picks up the flavor of white rice.

Tamarind. This is produced from the pulp of the hanging pod of the tamarind tree and has a fruity sweet-and-sour flavor. The most convenient form is in a bulk paste (instead of pods) which is sold in Indian or ethnic markets. It enhances the flavor of curry-based marinades and salad dressings.

Thyme. This aromatic herb imparts a rich, earthy flavor to food. With poultry, it's preferable to use fresh thyme; dried thyme only conveys its strength without its subtlety. It enhances the flavor of meat, poultry, fish, mushrooms and stuffing.

Turmeric. This root is a relative of ginger, and slightly deepens the flavors of vegetables and legumes. It also imparts a golden hue to dishes. Use in small amounts; too much will overpower food and can even make it taste bitter. Tumeric enhances the flavor of curries, chicken and sauces.

Vanilla. Obtained from the seed pod of a orchid, this flavoring agent is prized for its perfume and enhances the perception of sweet tastes.

COOKING FOR FLAVOR

Along with flavoring agents, cooking techniques can be used to enhance the flavor of foods. Barbecuing and smoking, caramelizing and steaming all enhance the natural flavors and textures of food without the addition of oil. Once you become familiar with these cooking methods, you'll never go back to frying and sautéing!

Caramelizing

This is one of the most important cooking techniques for creating flavorful low-fat cuisine. Caramelizing uses heat to convert starches to sugars, mellowing the flavor of foods that "bite." Use caramelized vegetables as a thickening agent to add "body" without the calories of oil.

Method 1

1. Heat a nonstick pan on medium heat until hot.
2. Add stock (fat removed), grated onions or garlic. Reduce heat to medium low, cover and sauté until soft, sweet and golden brown in color (about fifteen minutes).

Method 2

1. Preheat an oven to 300°. Place chopped onions or garlic in a roasting pan, and spray with nonstick vegetable spray (two-second spray).
2. Cook until soft (about thirty minutes).

DRY LOW-FAT COOKING METHODS

Barbecuing (Indirect Heat, Lid Closed)

This method uses a low circulating heat and smoke to cook the food. Although the cooking time is longer, the advantages of barbecuing are that the smoke imparts flavor and the meat remains moist. This method should be used for foods that require 25 minutes or more to cook (whole fish, roasts, chicken and turkey), fatty foods or those with flame-enhancing sugary marinades.

Barbecuing is my favorite method for cooking chicken. If you have a gas grill, set the temperature at 350° and place the breast bone side down. The skin is left on and removed before eating. Leaving the skin on keeps the meat moist so the chicken doesn't taste like cotton. Remove skin before eating.

Flavorful Smoke

You can enhance the flavor of barbecued food with wood chips and aromatic herbs, such as rosemary and fennel. If using wood, soak the chips in water for 30 minutes so that they will smoke rather than flame. Shake off excess water and place the chips on preheated charcoals for 2 minutes before adding food. If you're using a gas grill, place presoaked wood chips in a package of perforated tinfoil under the grill rack.

The best choices for smoking are:

Alder. Adds a subtle smoky flavor. Best used with oily fish, such as salmon and Chilean sea bass.

Fruitwoods. Impart subtle fruity flavors. The best choice for delicate fish.

Hickory. Imparts a bacony taste. Best suited to beef, chicken and lean pork.

Maple. Adds a subtle sweet tone. Works well with poultry.

Mesquite. Lends an earthy, woodsy taste. Use with meat, fish, seafood and poultry.

Oak. A mild relative of mesquite. Suited for poultry and fish.

Grilling and Health

Grilling is a healthy way of cooking. Only small amounts of oil are used during the cooking process to prevent drying and sticking of the meat to the grill. Additionally, most of the fat drips away rather than being reabsorbed into the food during cooking.

Although medical experts have voiced concern over the possibility of grilled foods increasing your risk of cancer, recent research has concluded that tons of nitrosomes (toxic chemical found in charred food) would have to be consumed on a daily basis before the effects are harmful.

Grilling (Direct Heat, Open Lid)

This cooking method uses direct heat—usually a fire—and the lid remains open. Grilling creates a hotter temperature than barbecuing, and produces foods that are crispy on the outside and juicy on the inside. An open grill should be used for foods that cook quickly, such as thin cuts of meat, fish fillets, shellfish, fruit and vegetables.

Fuel

Mesquite, oak and hickory lump charcoals start quicker, burn at a higher heat and won't leave an artificial chemical taste like charcoal briquettes. These hardwood charcoals should be used with meat, poultry, shellfish and dense fish. Alder, cherry and apple charcoals burn at a lower heat and seem to work better with the fragile fishes.

The easiest way to start a charcoal fire is by using a chimney starter or metal flue. Place crumbled pieces of newspaper into the bottom section and pile the charcoal directly on the grill to fill the top section to about three-fourths full. Set the flue on the grill's bottom and light the paper. The fire will spread to the charcoal and ignite it. The charcoals are ready to use when white in color (this takes about 30 minutes).

Gas

The advantages of using gas instead of charcoal are that the grill is ready to cook in only seven minutes, it's a less expensive fuel and clean-up is minimal.

Preparing the Grill

The grill is ready for cooking when the fire is no longer flaming. The temperature is "hot" when the coals are still red, and you can hold your hand at rack level for three seconds. A "moderate" temperature" is achieved when the coals are covered with a gray ash, and you can hold your hand at rack level for five to six seconds.

To prevent food from sticking to the grill, start with a clean grill (otherwise the food will catch on old pieces of burned-on food), preheat the grill for five minutes (food will stick to a cold grill) and lightly oil the rack before adding the foods.

Fish. Firm-fleshed fish such as salmon, mackerel, tuna, swordfish, halibut and monkfish are great candidates for grilling. Their dense flesh holds up well on the grill, and their higher fat content helps the flesh remain succulent. Fragile fish, such as sole and flounder, tend to dry out and fall apart. To prevent this from occurring, place a piece of heavy-duty perforated foil underneath the fish or put fish in a grill basket.

Fish should be room temperature before grilling. This allows the heat to penetrate to the center more quickly and prevents overcooking the outside. Coat fish with a mesquite, canola or olive oil spray (twice), and place fish perpendicular to the heated grill (rather than parallel) to minimize sticking.

There are two tests for checking if the fish is done. The first is to cut the fish in its thickest part—the flesh should just be losing its transparency. (Fish will continue to cook for a few minutes after it has been removed from the grill. If you remove it at this time, the flesh will be opaque throughout and moist when you serve it.

The second test is done by pressing the flesh—it should be firm but still spring back when touched.

The biggest mistake you can make when grilling is to move the fish before its protein is caramelized (the surface of the fish gets a "skin" or crust). This will cause the flesh to stick to the grill. For easy removal, slide a spatula under the fish in the *direction of the grill* and lift.

Seafood. Leave shrimp in the shell to retain moisture and flavor. The shellfish is done when the thickest part of the large tail end is turning opaque.

Vegetables. Grilled, marinated vegetables have a sweet, rich flavor that cannot be produced with any other cooking method.

The best vegetables for the grill are onions, mushrooms, squash, peppers and eggplant. Spray vegetables with a nonstick spray (mesquite, canola or olive oil), or baste with a marinade while grilling. A low-fat alternative is to wrap vegetables in banana, lettuce or cabbage leaves before grilling. The leaves will char without flaming and impart a subtle smoky flavor to the vegetables.

Grilling Guidelines

Grilling time is determined by the width of the food, temperature of the fire and distance of grill from the heat source. Since cooking times vary, do not mix different types of foods on the same skewer. You can enhance the flavor of grilled foods by marinating meat and poultry for three hours at room temperature, or six to twelve hours in the refrigerator before cooking. Fish and shellfish should be marinated for thirty minutes at room temperature, or two to three hours in the refrigerator before grilling.

Width	Method	Heat	Time	Distance from Fire
Fish (fillets)				
½ inch	direct	high	4–6 minutes	4 inches
¾ inch	direct	high	6–8 minutes	4 inches
1 inch	direct	high	10 minutes	4 inches
Whole Fish				
1–1½ inches				
(1–1½ lbs.)	indirect	low	12 minutes	4–6 inches
2–2½ inches				
(3–5 lbs.)	indirect	low	0–30 minutes	6 inches
3–5 inches				
(5–7 lbs.)	indirect	low	30–40 minutes	6 inches
Shellfish				
Clams (medium)	direct	moderate	4–6 minutes	4 inches
Crab (whole)	direct	moderate	10 minutes	4 inches
Lobster tail	direct	moderate	10 minutes	4 inches
Scallops (large)	direct	moderate	2 minutes	4 inches
Shrimp (large)	direct	moderate	4–6 minutes	4 inches
Chicken				
Whole	indirect	moderate	20 mins./pound	4 inches
Skinless breast	direct	high	8–12 minutes	4 inches
Turkey				
Whole	indirect	moderate	20 mins./pound	4 inches

Width	Method	Heat	Time	Distance from Fire
Turkey				
Skinless breast	direct	moderate	14–16 minutes	4 inches
Meat				
Veal (1½ inch)	direct	moderate-hot	7–8 minutes	4 inches
London broil	direct	moderate	5 minutes	4 inches
Vegetables (1-inch slice)				
eggplant	direct	low	5 minutes	4 inches
onion, peeled	direct	low	5 minutes	4 inches
mushrooms	direct	low	4–5 minutes	4 inches
tomatoes	direct	low	9–15 minutes	4 inches
(½-inch slice)				
Summer squash	direct	low	5–10 minutes	4 inches

Smoking

There are two methods for smoking foods: hot smoking and cold smoking. The difference between the two is time and temperature. Hot smoking (covered in barbecuing) takes several hours and uses a temperature of 200°, producing a firm texture that works well with poultry and meat.

Cold smoking takes a longer period of time (from hours to days) and uses temperatures that do not exceed 90°. The advantage of cold smoking is that it enhances, rather than conceals, the natural flavors of foods. When done correctly, cold smoking turns fish into a gourmet delight, imparting rich flavors and a succulent texture that melts in your mouth.

WET LOW-FAT COOKING METHODS

Microwaving

Produces good results in reheating foods and also cooking foods that have a high water content, such as vegetables and fish. The only bakery item that microwaves well is English muffins.

Poaching

Boiling a skinless, boneless chicken breast makes the meat dry and tasteless. You'll get a more tender and flavorful product if you simmer the meat for five to seven minutes, cover and set aside for an additional fifteen minutes to finish the cooking process. The secret to the success of this wet low-fat technique is using only enough liquid to cover the meat, which retains the chicken's flavor.

Steaming

Steaming uses gentle, moist heat from boiling liquids or water. It preserves the natural flavor and moisture of foods. This is a wonderful method for cooking fish, such as Chilean sea bass and salmon, or shellfish such as lobster, crab, shrimp or clams. Add herbs, ginger, garlic, chilies or scallions on top as an herbed crust, or stuff in the cavity if using a whole fish.

To add additional flavor while steaming, wrap the food in plant leaves such as lettuce, cabbage, banana, ti or avocado. Plant leaves work better than aluminum foil or corn husks because they impart a subtle flavor and also retain moisture better. You can find banana leaves at Oriental markets in the frozen food section. Ti leaves can be obtained at your local florist.

You'll get the best results with a Chinese bamboo steamer. The design prevents condensation that washes away taste. If you can't obtain one, wrap a towel around your pot lid to catch excess moisture. Herbs or spices can be added to the water to provide additional flavor. Lemongrass, tarragon, chilies, ginger, Old Bay Seasoning and garlic are some of my favorites.

Steam Frying

Add a few tablespoons of stock, wine or vinegar and cover food while frying in a nonstick pan on medium-low heat. This keeps food moist and produces a soft texture (will not produce a crust).

CHAPTER FOUR

NOT ALL CHILIES ARE CREATED EQUAL

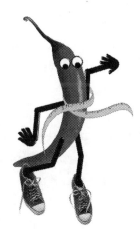

There are hundreds, perhaps thousands, of chilies in the world (and we'll learn about many of them in the next chapter). Classifying them is nearly impossible because the names they are known by vary from region to region. Further confusing the issue is the fact that chilies cross-pollinate easily, and new varieties are being discovered every day. However, all chilies known today originated from the indigenous South American plant, *Capsicum frutescens*.

Capsicums, which are from the Solanacae (nightshade) family, are botanically classified as a fruit. This fascinating fruit is in fact used as a vegetable, a spice and also a medicine. When harvested in its green stage—

after about 70 days—chilies are considered vegetables. Harvested fully ripened—after about 130 days—they are called a spice.

The biggest misconception about chilies is that they are simply hot. However, chilies have a tremendous range of flavors that include smoky, fruity, nutty, chocolatey and meaty. No other flavoring agent can offer such a wide range of tastes without expanding your waistline. Once you become familiar with the different types of chilies and how to use them, you won't want to eat food without them!

Flavor is linked to color, the majority of which is found in compounds in the flesh. For instance, a green chili is in an unripened state and usually has a tart, vegetable flavor, while a red chili is mature and has a sweeter, more complex flavor. This is caused, in part, by the increased sugar content and, in part, by the development of the carotenoid pigments, which reach their peak at maturity.

Fresh chilies are used as flavor accents, and when cooking with them, you must take into consideration their heat, tone and texture, all of which add character to a dish. Their mild flavor can be intensified by roasting; this transforms the "raw" vegetable tones to earthy, smoky flavors. One of the best ways to use roasted chilies is in a sauce—by blending two different varieties. With practice you'll be able to choose chilies whose flavors complement each other, such as poblanos and serranos, and combine them to add intricate dimensions in a dish.

Dried chilies make a bold statement—they define the flavor of a dish. The dehydration process intensifies a chili's flavor by condensing the oils and natural sugars, creating tastes that are rich and complex. In fact, different flavors and subtle tones emerge that were indiscernible in its fresh form. The most interesting way to use dried chilies is in combinations of two or three, which creates a harmony of hot, fruity and smoky flavors. For instance, blending chipotle, ancho and cascabel chilies creates a hot, smoky, raisin-flavored sauce with tones of an aged Bordeaux wine. Who needs béarnaise?

The aromas of chilies enhance their flavor. A chili's natural fragrance is produced by volatile oils, which are a mixture of esters, methoxypyrazies and aliphatic alcohols. The aliphatic alcohols and esters are responsible for the fruity and floral aromas, while smoky scents are created during the manufacturing process.

To use chilies with finesse, you must become familiar with their various aromas and use them to enhance the flavor of individual dishes. For instance, the habanero has a fruity fragrance that improves the taste of a mango salsa. The chipotle, which is a smoked jalapeno, has a smoky scent that enhances the flavor of chicken, meat or beans. Keep in mind that substituting chilies will change the character of a dish.

Capsicums contain a chemical, capsaicin, which gives this fruit its "heat." And, no two chilies are alike in this respect. Not only do different types of chilies produce variations in heat, but up to thirty-five different levels of piquancy can be obtained from the same plant! Recent research by Dr. Yayeh Zewdie found that chilies located on the lower branches, at the lower node positions of the plant, are the hottest.

Capsaicin is made up of elemental units called capsaicinoids, which are formed into a molecular chain. The "heat" comes from the arrangement of these molecules, which differ by the type of pepper. The perception of heat is felt when the chain is three or four carbons long but disappears when it reaches the eleventh (hottest range is at eight or nine carbon lengths).

Chilies exhibit tremendous variations in where they "bite." Jalapenos hit you in the back of the mouth; pasados produce a long, slow burn on the tongue; and habaneros sear your palate!

Where you feel the "heat" in your mouth is caused by the structure of the individual capsaicinoids. Researchers have identified twenty capsaicinoids that make up capsaicin: nordihydrocapsacin is the least irritating and has a fruity and sweet taste, dihydrocapsaicin causes a "rapid" bite, while homodihydrocapsaicin produces a prolonged burn on the tip of the tongue.

Capsaicin begins to develop around the fourth day of fruit development and is detectable by taste at two weeks. It reaches peak levels near the fruit's maturity, after which levels slowly decline during the ripening stage.

Additionally, the nutritional content of chilies changes with maturity. Green chilies, which are in an unripened state, contain high amounts of vitamin C (per gram weight, twice that of an orange). When chilies mature to red, they lose vitamin C, while at the same they time develop significant amounts of vitamin A. In fact, one tablespoon of red chili powder supplies the U.S.D.A. daily requirement for vitamin A. Moreover, all chilies are good sources of niacin, riboflavin, thiamine, magnesium, iron and phytochemicals. Phytochemicals, compounds found only in plants, have been linked to reduced oxidation of LDL, enhanced immune function and prevention of cancer.

Part of the Chili Pepper Diet is to get more familiar with this pungent pod.

WORKING WITH CHILIES

In Chicago, a man was admitted to a local emergency room complaining of severe pain. He had been preparing a large batch of chilies when he began to experience a burning sensation in his hands. Although he had not been exposed directly to a heat source, such as fire or hot water, he cried "his hands were on fire." The perplexed doctors finally diagnosed his condition as "Hunan hand"—a result of exposure to capsaicin.

When the nerve endings in your skin are irritated by capsaicin, they release stores of substance P, which is responsible for the burning sensation. Capsaicin initially stimulates and then blocks small-diameter pain fibers by depleting them of substance P. The stinging and burning sensation is called "sensitization," while the numbing effect is known as "desensitization," which occurs after repeated exposures. It is important to take precautionary measures when you are working with chilies to prevent the "shock" they produce. However, if you feel a burning sensation, don't panic. It is temporary, and should subside in fifteen to thirty minutes.

Chili Guidelines

1. Men should take precautions when working with chilies *before* urinating. Need I say more?
2. Be careful when working with chilies if you're going to handle a baby or change a baby's diapers.
3. *Never* handle chilies before you insert or remove contact lenses. Better yet, wear your glasses.
4. Protect your hands before you have sexual relations.
5. *Don't* handle chilies and touch your face after you've had a facial, wax treatments or used exfoliating agents.
6. When using a blender for pureeing chilies, remove the lid for a few seconds before putting your face over the chilies—the fumes can sting your eyes and nose.

How to Prevent "Hunan Hand"

1. Wear gloves (surgical gloves work the best because they don't impede the movement of your fingers). This is the most effective method for preventing a chili burn.
2. Apply a light coating of cooking oil to your hands.
3. Use a hand chopper for chopping fresh chilies and a spice grinder and scissors when preparing dry chilies.

How to Pick and Prepare Your Pods

Buying Fresh Chilies

Select chilies that are firm, dry and heavy for their size. The skin should be shiny, smooth and unblemished.

Storing Fresh Chilies

Wash chilies to remove dirt, then dry them and wrap them in paper towels to absorb excess moisture, which hastens the spoiling process. Store wrapped chilies in the crisper section of the refrigerator, where they should keep for two or three weeks.

To extend their shelf life, remove the chilies from the refrigerator every four or five days and dry them off with a paper towel. Return them to their storage container. Do not store fresh chilies in a plastic bag— moisture will accumulate and hasten the spoiling process. It is possible to store peppers in a resealable plastic bag, provided all air is expelled to prevent spoilage. This can be done by sucking out the air with a straw.

Do not leave chilies out in the open for extended periods of time—

they will rapidly lose flavor and texture. However, if you intend to use them within a short period, you can keep them in a paper bag.

Roasting and Peeling

When you roast green chilies and remove the skin (which has a bitter flavor), their green vegetable taste is transformed to a smoky, earthy flavor. Always make a small hole or a slit in the chili to vent gas, which prevents explosions (shooting seeds can travel five to six feet and are *painful* if they get in your eyes).

Step 1: Roasting

Broiler: Preheat the broiler. Arrange the peppers on a broiler pan and place three to five inches under the broiler. Turn the pods until completely charred. (If you need a firm texture in the peppers, do not use a broiler, which can overcook them. However, if you are using the peppers in a sauce, chowder or stew, this is a wonderful technique.)

Electric stove: Set the burner on high and place a cooling rack over the coil. Place the chilies on the rack, and rotate them with kitchen tongs as they blacken and blister until the all sides of the peppers have charred. Never let the skin of the chili touch the electric coil, and remove the peppers immediately when charred.

Gas stove: The best way to roast a large chili is directly over a gas flame on the stove. Set the flame on medium and place the chilies on the burner trivet. As the skin blackens and blisters, rotate the chili with kitchen tongs to cook evenly.

Grilling: Preheat the grill on high. Place the pepper on a rack and turn as it blisters, until the entire pepper is charred.

Oven roasting: Preheat the oven to 550°. Arrange the peppers on a rack until blistered (three to seven minutes). Turning is not required.

Skillet: Preheat a heavy cast-iron skillet or griddle on medium-high heat until hot. Put the pepper in the skillet and turn as it blisters, until the entire pepper is charred. Split the roasted, peeled chili open and scoop out the seeds and membranes with the tip of a knife. Roasted and peeled chilies will keep in the refrigerator for up to two days.

Step 2: Removing Skin

After the skin is blistered, the chili must be steamed to remove the skin. Various methods of steaming "lifts" the skin, which makes it easy to remove without tearing the flesh.

Towel: After roasting the chili, wrap it with a cool, moist kitchen towel and allow to cool (ten to twenty minutes). This the most reliable method for removing the skin.

Ice water: Plunge the chili into ice water. The advantage of this method is that it produces a crisper pod because it stops the cooking process immediately. The disadvantage is that it washes away some of the oils that give the chili its flavor. Do not use this method with a poblano—it removes that chili's wonderful smoky flavor!

Bag: Place in a paper or plastic bag for fifteen minutes. Although some people have luck with this method, I don't. The skin will often stick to the flesh, and the chili ends up being torn.

Step 3: Peeling

Once the chili has cooled, it can be easily peeled off with your fingers. I find this a more reliable method than using a knife, which frequently tears the skin.

Step 4: Peeling (to Reduce Heat in Chili)

Slit the chili, and either remove the seeds and veins with your fingers or scoop them out with a small spoon, which will reduce the heat of a chili. Do not wash the roasted, peeled chili or place under running water—this will dilute the oils that give it flavor!

PRESERVING PEPPERS

Freezing

Freezing is a good way to preserve fresh chilies: You'll have an ample supply in the winter months, when they are more difficult to obtain. Although they will retain their heat and flavor, you can expect them to lose their crisp texture because of cell wall rupture. Because oxygen destroys vitamin C, as long as you do not expose the peeled pod to air, you will retain most of its nutritive value. Leaving the charred skin on a roasted pepper before you freeze it will help prevent the loss of vitamin C.

Large chilies (Anaheim, poblano, New Mexico):

1. Individually wrap the cooled, blistered chili in plastic wrap (skin will easily come off when the pod is thawed).
2. Freeze the entire pod to prevent loss of vitamin C.
3. Place in heavy-duty (freezer) resealable plastic bags, expressing as much air as possible.

Small chilies (serranos, jalapenos, japones, arbols, etc.):

1. Wash peppers.
2. Dry peppers.
3. Separate peppers and place them on a metal pan (this prevents them from sticking together).
4. Freeze.
5. When frozen, place the peppers in a freezer (heavy-duty) resealable bag, removing as much air as possible.
6. Return to the freezer and use as needed. Can be kept for twelve months.

Drying

Sun-Drying

This ancient method was used by the Native Americans to preserve chilies for use in the winter months. The disadvantage of this method is that sunlight will diminish both vitamin C and capsaicin content. Try it only if you live in a dry climate.

Green, thick-skinned chilies (serrano, poblano, etc.):

1. Wash chilies.
2. Peel chilies.

3. Remove seeds and veins.
4. Spread chilies on a rack in a single layer.
5. Cover with a cheesecloth to protect from insects and birds.
6. Place the rack in the sun and turn occasionally.
7. Bring chilies in at night to prevent spoilage from moisture. (Process usually takes two days.)

Red, thin-skinned chilies (guajillo, New Mexico, etc.):

1. Put the chilies (whole) on a rack and place in the sun.
2. Cover with a cheesecloth to protect from insects and birds.
3. Bring in at night to prevent spoilage from moisture. (Process takes five to six days.)

On the plant:

1. Cut chili at bottom of stem.
2. Tie a string to stem (at the bottom).
3. Hang upside down in the sun (should not touch other plants; needs air circulation to dry properly).
4. Bring in at night to prevent spoilage from moisture. (Process takes about seven to fourteen days.)

Oven-Drying

This is a good technique for preserving thin-skinned green chilies. It helps retain vitamin C since the peppers aren't exposed to sunlight.

1. Roast peppers.
2. Peel peppers.
3. Remove seeds and veins.
4. Cut in three-quarter-inch strips.
5. Preheat oven to 140°.

6. Set on racks, and turn every four hours.

7. Leave the oven door slightly open to allow moisture to escape. (Takes eight hours for thin-skinned peppers; ten hours for thicker-skinned peppers.)

Pickling

Pickled peppers are eaten in Mexico as an appetizer. Frequently, sliced raw carrots, onions and garlic are added.

1. Pierce the jalapeno or serrano chilies (about one-half pound) several times with a toothpick to allow the marinade to penetrate. (Pickling seems to work best with fresh green chilies. Don't mix the peppers; otherwise the flavors will blend.)

2. Heat one tablespoon of corn oil in a heavy twelve-inch nonstick pan on medium heat. Add one cup of sliced onion, one peeled, sliced carrot, and five cloves of garlic, stirring until the onion is tender. Add chilies and cook until the chilies begin to soften (about five minutes).

3. Add one cup of a vinegar (rice wine vinegar or distilled vinegar) and one-half cup water to the vegetable mixture, and bring to a boil. Reduce heat to low, cover and simmer for five minutes. Remove from heat, and cool.

4. Fill a sterile glass jar with chilies and vegetable mixture.

5. Add two teaspoons of Mexican oregano; five black peppercorns; one teaspoon kosher salt; three dried juniper berries and one bay leaf.

6. Cover with equal parts of water and vinegar if chilies are not submerged.

7. Place in refrigerator for two days. Keeps for two weeks if chilies are completely submerged in vinegar.

DRIED CHILIES

Buying Dried Chilies

Fresh chilies have a good aroma, brilliant color and pliable texture; old peppers are faded and brittle. A simple test for freshness is if you can gently bend them back and forth without breakage. Discard any broken chilies, because the volatile oils that carry the flavors evaporate when exposed to air. Your best bet is to buy unpackaged chilies in Latin or Oriental markets, where they have a quick turnover rate and the stock remains fresh. A good alternative is buying chilies directly from wholesalers (the best ones I found are listed later in this book).

Storage

If stored properly, dried peppers stay fresh for up to six months. The best storage containers are glass or plastic jars. Keep dried peppers in a cool, dark place, preferably in a closed kitchen cabinet. If you store chilies in a freezer, check them at least once a month for signs of mildew, which usually starts around the seeds (allow the pods to come to room temperature before using).

When improperly stored, dried peppers are subject to bug infesta.tion. If you find a powdery dust around the peppers or tiny holes in the skin, break open the peppers and look for insects. The most common pest is the corn moth, which looks like a small worm in its larvae stage and changes to a small flying moth at maturity. If the chili wholesaler has kept the peppers near infested flour or corn meal, you'll have a problem in about three weeks.

Powders

Dried chili can be made into a powder by pulverizing it in a spice or electric coffee grinder. Powders are a wonderful form of chili to use in soups, salsas or any dish where the chili needs to be dissolved. Buy a separate electric coffee grinder for dried chilies; the hot, volatile oils contained in chilies stick to the grinding blade, which would turn your morning coffee into "jet fuel."

Here's how to prepare chili powder:

1. Remove stems, seeds and veins of four to five small chilies.
2. Break into little pieces (if chili is large).
3. Place chili in a grinder.
4. Cup the grinder with both hands (thumbs on top and fingers curled around the sides).
5. Shake the grinder in an up-and-down motion while grinding (about five to ten seconds) until pulverized. You should stop every ten seconds, shake and regrind.
6. Remove and sift out larger pieces. Regrind until a coarse powder is formed.
7. Store chili powder in a glass jar in a cool, dark place.

NOTE: One tablespoon of dried ancho, pasilla or mulato chili is equal to one whole dried chili; one-eighth of a teaspoon is equal to one whole àrbol, cayenne or Thai chili.

Toasting

Toasting dried chilies further intensifies the flavor. Heat releases the oils, which amplifies its more subtle tones. For instance, when you toast an ancho chili, you'll initially experience a smoky taste on the back of your tongue. It's followed by a fruity flavor—usually plum, raisin or cherry—in the middle of your tongue. It finishes with a kiss of chocolate on your tongue's tip. Chefs call this "mouth surfing." You'll call it heaven.

Pan-fry

1. Heat a heavy cast-iron skillet or griddle until hot.
2. Place a few chilies in a pan until you smell a fragrance and turn (two or three seconds on each side). Be careful not to scorch the dried chili because the oils in the pod will take on a acrid and bitter taste.

Gas stove

1. Set the gas flame on a stove on high.
2. Hold the chili by the stem and place over the flame for a few seconds, turning back and forth until fragrant (three to four seconds on each side). Be careful not to hold the chili over the flame for too long—it will take on a bitter taste and cannot be used.

TIP: Do not try to toast a dried chili with a cigarette lighter; it will absorb the flavor of the lighter fluid and not be suitable for use.

Rehydration

Unless you are using a powder or flakes, dried chilies should be plumped up with water before adding to recipes.

1. Simmer water in a pan.
2. Place the chilies in the hot water, cover, and remove from heat.
3. Let stand for twenty minutes.
5. Remove the chili from water and allow to cool.
6. Remove stem, seeds and veins. The chili is now ready for use—either by chopping, shredding or pureeing—in soups or sauces. (Thin-skinned chilies, such as guajillos, should be slit open and the pulp scraped out with a spoon.)

TIP: Save the flavored soaking liquid for use in soups, sauces and bean spreads.

Making a Paste

Pastes are great way to add both flavor and texture to sauces, soups or nonfat mayonnaise. They should be stored in the refrigerator, in a glass container (plastic containers will absorb the color of the paste).

Cold method

1. Remove stem and seeds from chilies.
2. Cover dried chilies with cold water for twenty-four hours (hot water leeches some of the flavor).
3. Add chilies and one teaspoon of kosher salt to a coffee grinder and blend till smooth. You can also use a mortar.

Hot method

1. Cover chili with hot water for twenty minutes.
2. Remove stem, seeds and break chili into pieces.
3. Place in a electric coffee grinder or use a hand-held blender and puree.

Pepper Sauces

In New Orleans, I found over ninety different hot sauces from around the world. Basically, sauces fall into three categories: whole chilies preserved in brine or vinegar, fermented pureed chilies and pureed chilies. Sauces come in varying degrees of heat and flavor. Some provide mostly heat, while others are blended with tomatoes, spices and tropical fruits to provide more flavor.

Powdered Chili

The commercial chili powders commonly found in markets are a mixture of 40 percent chilies (ancho and New Mexico) and 60 percent spices and corn flour, which are added to extend the product. Avoid these commercially prepared products because the flavor of the chili is either diluted or changed. Add your own oregano, cumin or garlic to suit the individual recipe.

CHAPTER FIVE

CHILIES: ALL THE WAY FROM HOT TO MILD

There are neon orange habaneros, bumpy green poblanos, and glossy red Thais that look like lacquered fingernails. Heart-shaped anchos smell like raisins, while smoky chipotles impart a rich, haunting note to sauces. Some chilies tickle your tongue, while others induce a baptism by fire.

No other vegetable—or food for that matter—has made such a dramatic impact in the culinary world. Although garlic and chocolate have attained celebrity status (and cult followings), chilies have emerged as the superstar of the über-foods. And there's a good reason for this: Chilies not only seduce your palate with flavor, they thrill it with heat.

Spices and herbs tease low-fat dishes into something interesting. Chilies are your taste buds' wake-up call. What is special about chilies is capsaicin, the alkaloid that produces a pepper's heat. This tasteless, odorless chemical adds a new dimension to the culinary equation by tickling the nerves in your tongue, throat and palate. Agitated, these nerves send a message to your brain that your mouth is on fire. Your brain races to douse the pain by releasing endorphins, which trigger a rush of exquisite relief. Chilies transform eating into an exhilarating experience.

Capsicums are the consummate culinary tool that make it easy to reduce the amount of fat, sugar and salt in your diet. Chilies layer flavors—different flavors are sensed in different parts of the tongue and palate at different times—which makes the food we taste enticing. For instance, the citrus notes are sensed by the sour receptors along the sides, while the slightly bitter, dark chocolate tone of an ancho is tasted on the back of the tongue. The heat acts as the modulation in the flavor aria—it grabs your attention. A chili's complex flavors, heightened by heat, create a symphony of tastes that transport your low-fat food into the realm of the sublime.

MEASURING THE HEAT

In 1912, chemist Wlbur Scoville developed a taste-dilution test to measure the heat of peppers. Named after its inventor, the Scoville Organoleptic Test involved mixing pure chili powder with a sugar-water solution that was tasted by a panel of testers, in increasingly diluted concentrations, until they could no longer detect a burning sensation. Specific chilies were then assigned a number that reflected the amount of dilution required before the sensation of heat could no longer be perceived.

Over time, Scoville's test proved too inaccurate for the food industry to rely on. Alarming differences in test results emerged because results were based on subjective judgments. Although Scoville units remain the food industry's standard of measurement for hotness, the Scoville Organoleptic Test has been replaced by computerized technology. Today, the precise heat of a chili is measured using a process called high-pressure liquid chromatography (HPLC). The results of this test are converted into Scoville units: the hotter the chili, the higher the number of units.

The Scoville scale measures a pepper's heat in multiples of 100 units, ranging from cool bell peppers at zero to incendiary habaneros topping the chart at 300,000 units. Pure capsaicin registers at 16,000,000.

Currently, this scale is being updated to include hotter peppers. Chemists recently tested a new variety of habanero, Red Savina, that rated over 577,000 units! Today, breeders claim they will beat this shattering record with the upcoming Francisca habanero.

A simplified scale of 1 (mildest) to 10 (hottest) is also used to assign heat levels to a variety of peppers. Though not as precise, this modified version is easier to use. It is important to note that all heat scales are a general guideline, and variances in levels will occur because of a variety of growing conditions.

What's Hot, What's Not?

Heat	Scoville Units	Chilies & Condiments	Comments
	577,000	Red Savina habanero	Thermo-nuclear
	210,000	Red habanero	
	150,000	Orange habanero	
	200,000–577,000	Habanero	
10	100,000–350,000	Scotch bonnet, Thai, African "birds eye"	Incendiary; takes your breath away
9	50,000–100,000	Chilitepin, rocoto	Blistering
8	30,000–50,000	Pequin, cayenne, Tabasco, Chinese	Searing Sweat-inducing
7	15,000–30,000	De àrbol, crushed red pepper	Combustion Nose runs
6	5,000–15,000	Serrano, morita	Sizzling Body heats up
5	2,500–5,000	Jalapeno, chipotle	Stinging
4	1,500–2,500	Cascabel, Yellow Hot Wax, Guajillo, cherry	Singeing
3	1,000–1,500	Ancho, pasilla, pasado	Smoldering
2	500–1,000	Mulato, poblano, New Mexico	Warm, mellow heat
1	100–500	canned green chilies, Hungarian paprika (hot)	Tickles tongue
	10–100	pickled pepperoncini	Lukewarm
0		Bell peppers, U.S. paprika	No heat

In this chart, I have subjectively described what these numbers mean.

FRESH CHILIES

HABANERO

(ah-bah-*neh*-ro)

Comes from the Caribbean coast of Mexico (Yucatan region), land of the Mayans. Remove the seeds before using in a recipe.

Appearance: Orange, red, white and purple. Looks like a small Chinese lantern or mini bell pepper.

Heat: 10 to off the charts. Hottest of all chilies! Produces an incendiary heat that takes your breath away.

Taste: When fresh, has a tropical fruit flavor that is a blend of mango and pineapple with heat. Dried, the habanero loses its fruit flavor and is used primarily for heat.

Uses: Salsas, fish, seafood—especially shrimp, scallops and lobster—and table sauces.

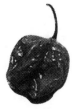

MANZANA

(mahn-*zah*-na)

In Spanish, name translates to "apple," which describes its round shape. This exquisite chili is unusual in that it has black seeds. Commonly used in western and central Mexican cuisine. Also known as chili caballo, chili rocoto and chili peron.

Appearance: Yellow-orange in color. Looks like a small bell pepper—3 inches long, 2¼ to 3 inches wide.

Heat: 6 to 8.

Taste: Mild fruitiness with a searing heat. Flavor resembles a yellow bell pepper, although not as sweet. Has a thin skin and a meaty texture.

Uses: Salsas, sauces and kebabs. It can be sliced into thin strips and added to other dishes, such as tuna fajitas.

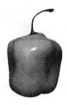

SERRANO

(seh-*rah*-no)

In Spanish, denotes the site of cultivation; specifically "in the mountains" (in northern Pueblo and Hidalgo, Mexico). The best green chili to use in tomato-based salsas.

Appearance: Light-green when immature. Red, orange or red-brown when mature. Column shaped; 1 to 2 inches long, ½-inch wide.

Heat: 6.

Taste: Full-bodied flavor with an acidic edge. Reds are sweeter. Flavor becomes more rounded with roasting.

Uses: Fresh: salsas, ceviches. Roasted: sauces.

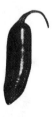

JALAPENO

(hal-*lah*-pay-no)

Name refers to its site of origin: Jalapa, Mexico. The most widely available green chili in the United States.

Appearance: Green, with vertical tan lines, when immature. Bright red when mature. Triangular-shaped, with rounded tip; 2 to 3 inches long, 1½ inches wide.

Heat: 5 to 6. Mexican jalapenos tend to be hotter than chilies grown in California.

Taste: Full-bodied flavor. Red jalapenos have a sweeter taste. Produces a sharp sting that is felt in the back of the mouth and throat. Available pickled (*en escabeche*); the pickling juice imparts a pleasant tartness that balances the heat. Use Mexican brands of pickled jalapenos—U.S. versions are too vinegary, and have an acrid taste. (Mexican brands of pickled jalapenos can be ordered at *http://www.monterreyfood products.com.*)

Uses: Salsas, soups, salads, sauces, breads and beans. Substitute a Dutch red chili if the red jalapeno is out of season.

GUËRO

(ge-where-o)

In Spanish, name means blonde, referring to its light yellow color. Has a wide range of heat; some have no heat, while others hit 8 on the heat scale. Also known as a wax pepper.

Appearance: Light yellow when immature. Red when ripe. Triangular-shaped; 4 inches long and 2 inches wide.

Heat: 5 to 8.

Taste: Slightly sweet with a waxy taste. Watery taste is improved with roasting.

Uses: Salads, sauces. Frequently pickled.

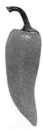

POBLANO

(po-*blah*-no)

Often mistaken for the pasilla chili, especially in California. Poblanos must be roasted, then peeled before using in a recipe—never eaten fresh. This process removes their tough skins, and develops a smoky flavor. When buying poblanos, choose the largest chilies—they are easier to roast and have a richer flavor.

Appearance: Dark green with a black tint. Resembles an elongated, bumpy bell pepper in shape; 4 to 5 inches long and 2½ to 3 inches wide.

Heat: 2.

Taste: Smoky, rich green vegetable flavor.

Uses: Sauces, soups and rice. Exceptional for enhancing the flavor of red meat.

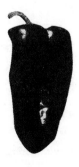

DRIED CHILIES

CAYENNE

(ki-yen)

Used in Creole cooking.

Appearance: Red. Primarily used in powdered form.

Heat: 8.

Taste: Has a tart, acidic flavor with dusty tones. Used more for heat than flavor.

Uses: Sauces and soups.

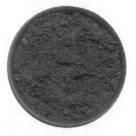

PEQUIN

(pe-*keen*)

Similar to the fiery fruit discovered by Christopher Columbus. Grows in the Southwest, Mexico, Central and South America. Not as blistering as its wild cousin, chilitepin. Also known as chili pequeno.

Appearance: Orange-red color. Oval shape resembles a large peppercorn; about ½ to ¾ inches long and ¼-inch wide.

Heat: 8. Produces an intense, stinging heat that dissipates quickly.

Taste: Delicate, smoky flavor with tones of citrus and corn.

Uses: Salsas, soups, beans, lentils and vinegars. In powder form with fruits and corn on the cob.

CHILI DE ÀRBOL

(day-ar-*bowl*)

In Spanish, translates to "tree chili." In Mexico, this chili is frequently used in "cooked" table salsas. A close cousin to cayenne.

Appearance: Bright reddish-brown color. Slender, bullet-shaped with a pointed tip; 2 to 3 inches long and ¼- to ⅜-inch wide.

Heat: 7 to 8. Produces a burning, acidic heat felt on the tip of the tongue.

Taste: Delicate, smoky flavor with tones of tannin. Provides more heat than flavor.

Uses: Salsas, soups, beans and vinegars. In powder form with sauces.

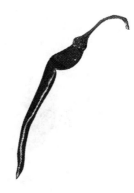

MORITA

(mor-*ee*-tah)

In Spanish, name translates to "little blackberry." A variety of dried, smoked red jalapeno. Has a sweeter, hotter flavor than the chipotle.

Appearance: Ruby-red with a brown cast. Triangular shape; 1 to 2 inches long and ⅜-inch wide.

Heat: 6 to 7.

Taste: Complex. Begins with a hot, smoky-sweet flavor in the back of the tongue; builds to a plum flavor on the middle; and finishes with a lingering tobacco taste on the tip. Imparts a ham flavor to food.

Uses: Meat, chicken, beans, sauces, salsas and soups.

NEW MEXICO

(Green)

Roasted, peeled and dried form of New Mexico or California chili.

Appearance: Olive to dark-green in color. Flat and tapered; measures 4 to 5 inches long, 1 inch wide.

Heat: 2 to 7.

Taste: Has a delicate, smoky, slightly sweet flavor with tones of citrus and celery.

Uses: Soups, stews and jerky.

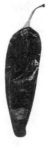

NEW MEXICO
(Red)

The quintessential soul-satisfying, comfort-food chili. Key ingredient that forms the backdrop in traditional Mexican and Southwestern red chili sauces. It is sweetened by roasted garlic and becomes darkly rich in the presence of cumin. Also known as Chili Colorado and Chili California.

Appearance: Bright red-brick color. Elongated and tapered; measures 5 to 7 inches long, 1½ to 2 inches wide.

Heat: 2 to 4. Produces a warm, mellow heat.

Taste: Acts as the "bass note" in a dish; adds depth and does not overwhelm. Deep, earthy flavor, with a slightly acidic edge and hint of sage.

Uses: Sauces and soups.

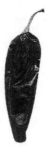

CHIPOTLE

(chi-*poat*-lay)

Dried, smoked, red jalapeno pepper. Flavor varies with type of smoking agent—mesquite, fruit trees, hardwoods or peat. Many consider mesquite wood the best smoking agent—it imparts a more smoky taste and richer flavor.

Appearance: Tobacco brown with tan veining; 2 to 4 inches long, ½-inch wide.

Heat: 5 to 6.

Taste: Intense, smoky finishing with a slightly sweet, subtle tobacco flavor. Tastes and smells like bacon.

Uses: Beans, soups, sauces, corn dishes, poultry, meat, salad dressings and condiments.

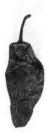

GUAJILLO

(gwa-*hee*-o)

In Spanish, name translates to "little gourd." This is one of the most popular chilies in Mexico. It has a very distinct flavor, and small amounts add both color and flavor to the dishes prepared with them.

Appearance: Reddish brown in color. Elongated and triangular-shaped; 5 inches long, 1 inch wide.

Heat: 4.

Taste: First earthy, then citrus with a sweet heat. Has tones of green tea and tannin with fruity aroma.

Uses: Salsas, sauces, soups and seafood—especially shrimps and scallops.

ANCHO

(*an*-choe)

Dried red poblano chili. Ancho, meaning "wide" in Spanish, is descriptive of its unique "broad-shouldered" shape. Famous for its use in the preparation of Mexican mole sauce.

Appearance: Purple-black color. Wrinkled skin and wide shoulder; 4 to 5 inches long, 3 inches wide. Rehydrates red.

Heat: 3 to 5.

Taste: Spicy, hot raisin with tones of dark chocolate. Sweetest of all the dried chilies. Flavor intensifies when the chili is toasted, amplifying chocolate tones.

Uses: Salsas, sauces, soups and fruit.

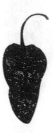

PASILLA

(pa-*see*-ah)

Name translates to "little raisin"—a dried form of the chilaca chili. Many times confused with the ancho chili, especially in California. Can be distinguished from the ancho when held up to light by its brown-black color; an ancho is red-brown in color.

Appearance: Dark, raisin-brown color. Shaped like a plump, curved Chinese green bean; 6 to 12 inches long and 1 inch wide.

Heat: 3 to 5.

Taste: Tastes like berries, with a slash of chocolate.

Uses: Best used in combination with other chilies in sauces, soups or stews. Enhances the flavor of seafood and chicken. Exquisite when used with anchos and guadillos.

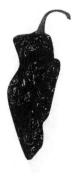

CASCABEL

(cas-*ka*-bell)

Means "rattle" in Spanish, which it resembles with its round shape when it's shaken (loose seeds produce a rattling sound).

Appearance: Reddish-brown in color. Shaped like a ball; 1 inch in diameter.

Heat: 4.

Taste: Has a woodsy, nutty flavor with tones of berry. Similar to an aged Bordeaux wine. The nutty flavor is intensified when it's dried, then toasted.

Uses: Ceviche, salsas, broths and sauces. In powder form with corn dishes and soups.

PASADO
(pa-*sah*-do)

A New Mexico red chili that has been dried, roasted and peeled. A favorite chili of the Pueblo Indians, who use them in winter when fresh chilies are no longer available.

Appearance: Orange-red color. Long, triangular shape; 4 inches long, 1 inch wide.

Heat: 3 to 4. Produces a lingering heat felt on the tip of the tongue.

Taste: Slightly sweet and smoky flavor with tones of toasted apple and cherry.

Uses: Soups and breads.

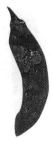

MULATO

(moo-*lah*-toe)

A variety of the dried poblano chili. Part of the "Holy Trinity" of chilies (ancho, pasilla and mulato). Has a richer chocolate flavor compared to the ancho.

Appearance: Chocolate-brown. Triangular shape with rounded shoulders tapering to a point. About 5 inches long and 2 to 3 inches wide. Rehydrates brown.

Heat: 2 to 4.

Taste: Complex. Starts smoky, builds to a fruity raisin flavor, crests to chocolate and finishes with a splash of tobacco.

Uses: Soups, sauces and salsas.

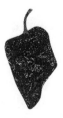

CHILI PEPPER GUIDE

Anaheim or Chipotle?
Manzana or Thai?

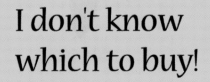

I don't know
which to buy!

Chili Pepper Guide: Contents

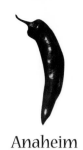
Anaheim

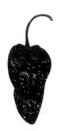
Ancho

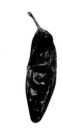
California

Cascabel

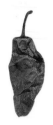
Chipotle

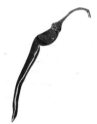
De Àrbol

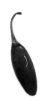
Dried Red Serrano

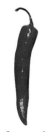
Dutch Red Chili

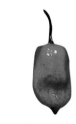
Fresh Habanero

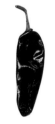
Guajillo

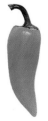
Guëro

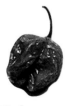
Habanero

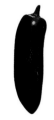
Jalapeno

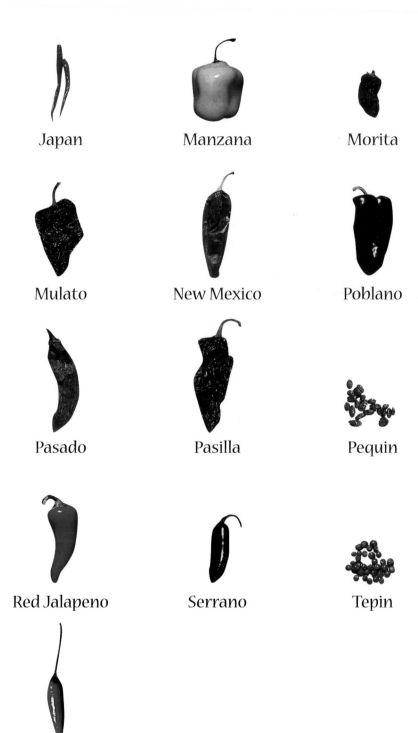

Japan

Manzana

Morita

Mulato

New Mexico

Poblano

Pasado

Pasilla

Pequin

Red Jalapeno

Serrano

Tepin

Thai

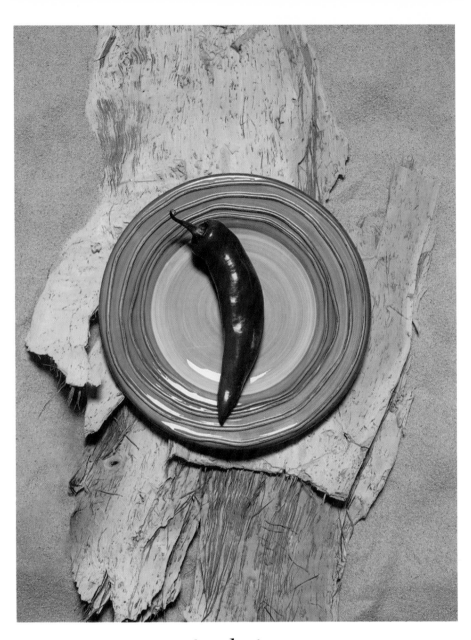

Anaheim

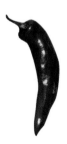

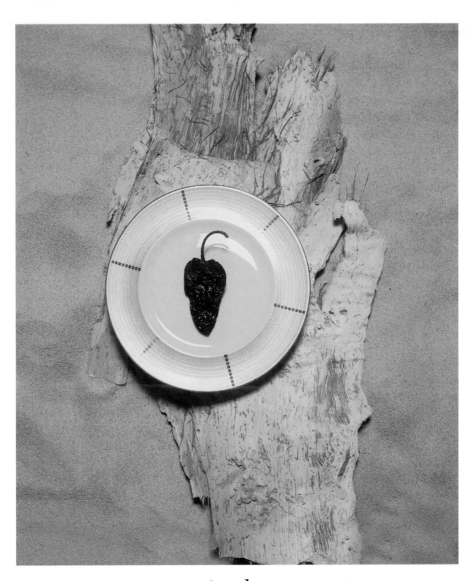

Ancho

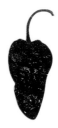

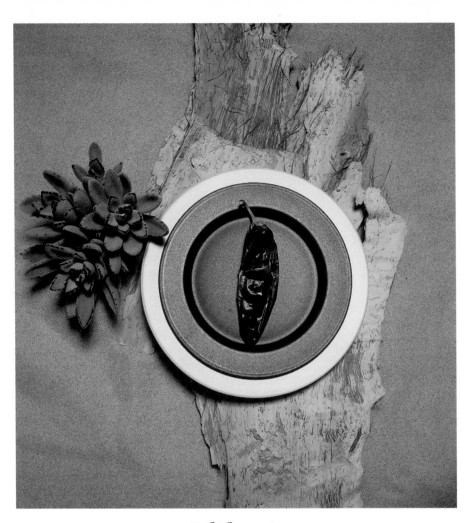

California

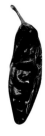

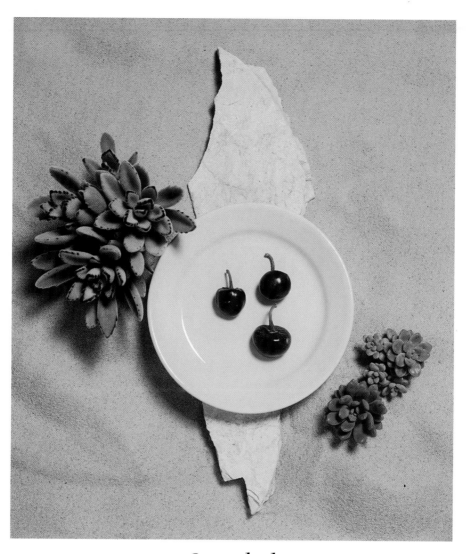

Cascabel

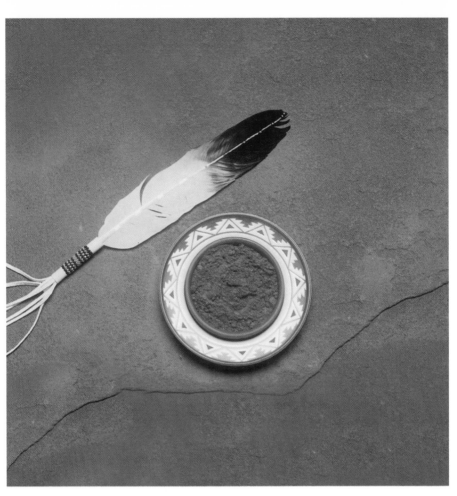

Cayenne Powder

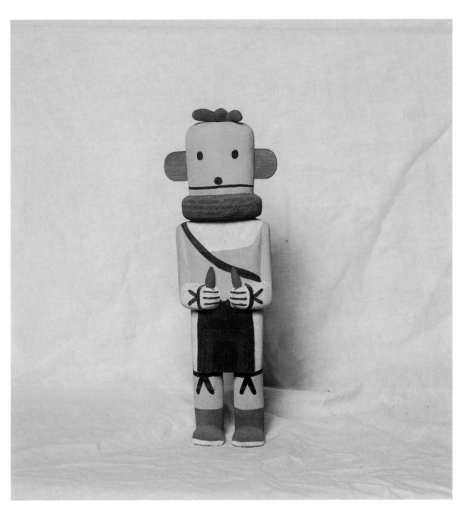

Chili Katchina

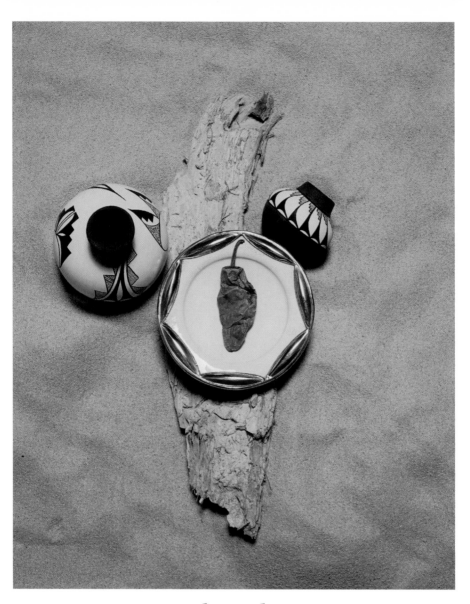

Chipotle

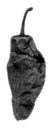

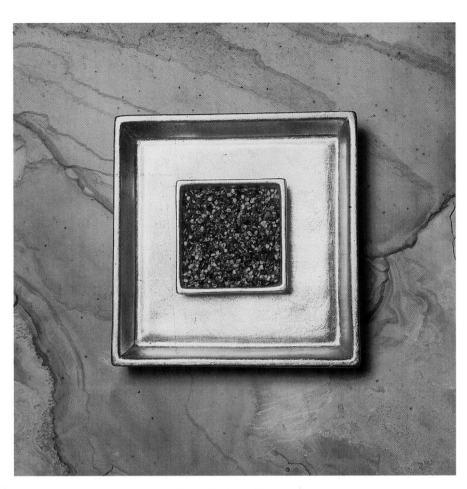

Crushed Red Pepper

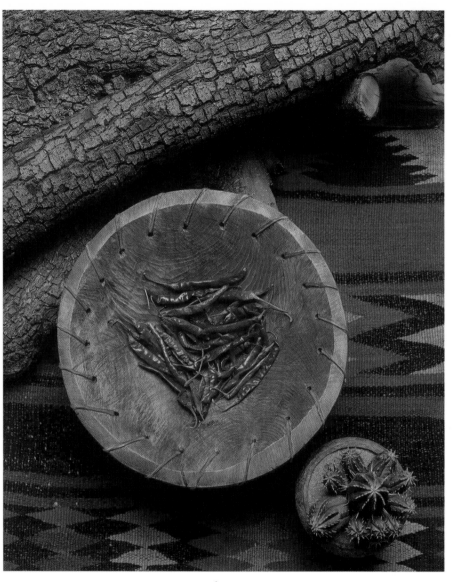

De Àrbol

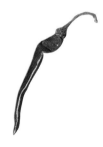

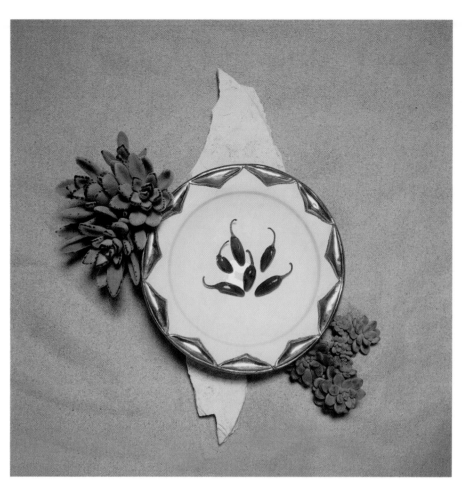

Dried Red Serrano

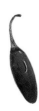

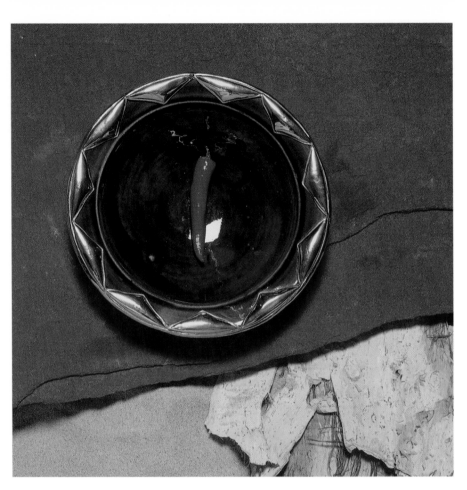

Dutch Red Chili

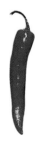

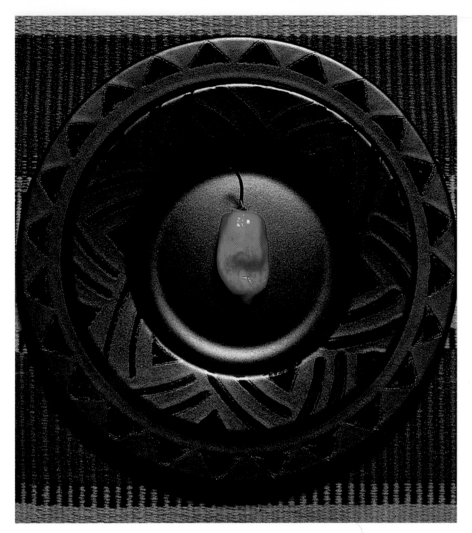

Fresh Habanero

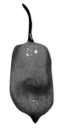

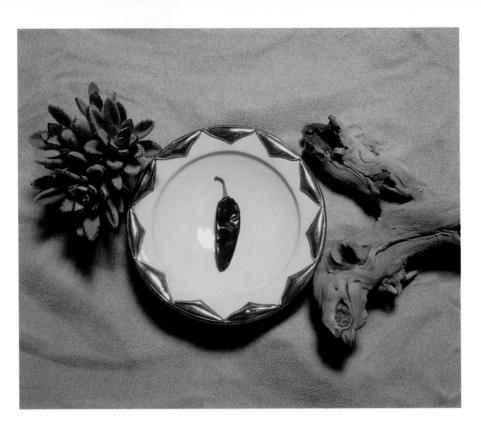

Guajillo

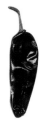

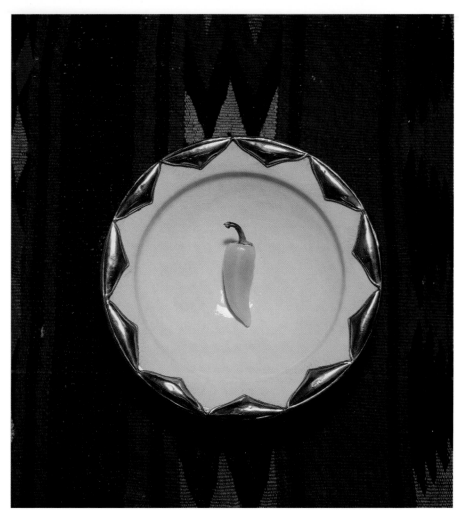

Guëro

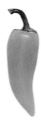

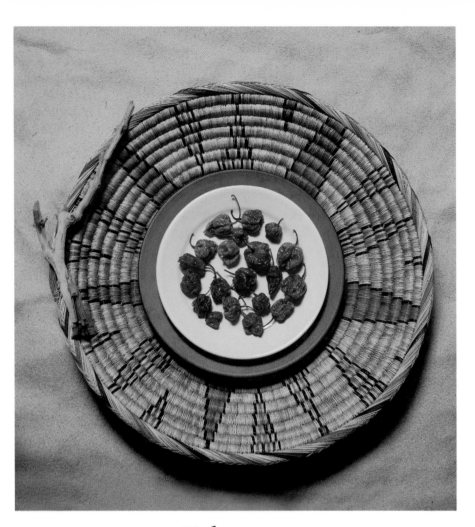

Habanero

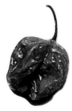

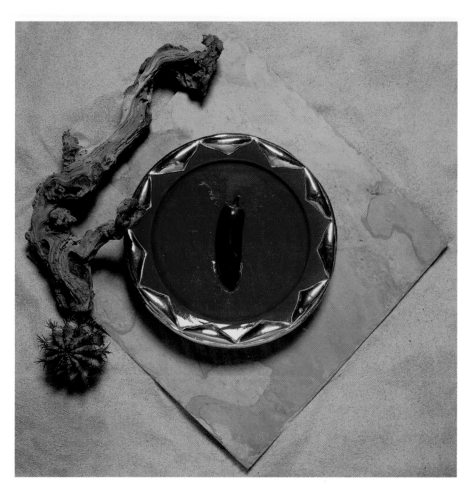

Jalapeno

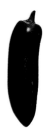

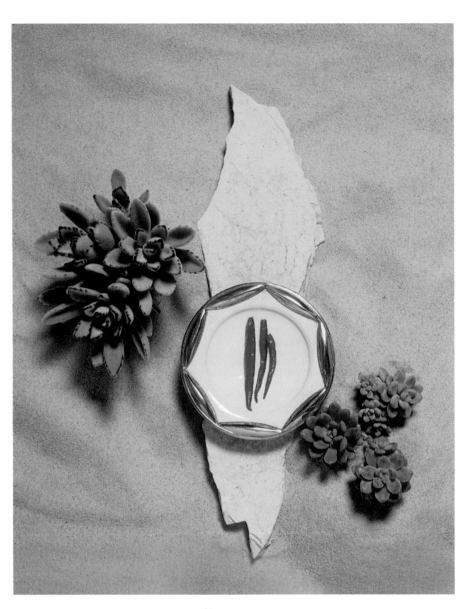

Japan

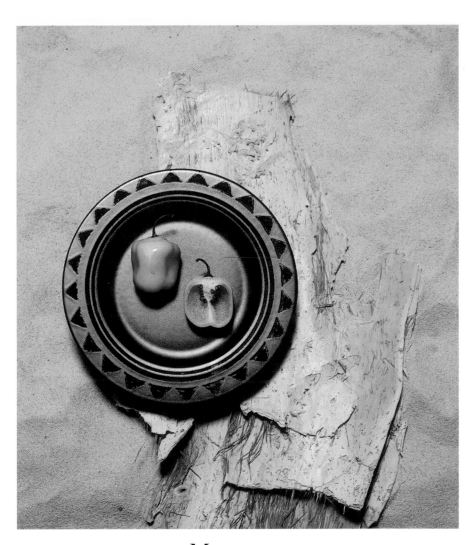

Manzana

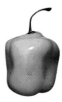

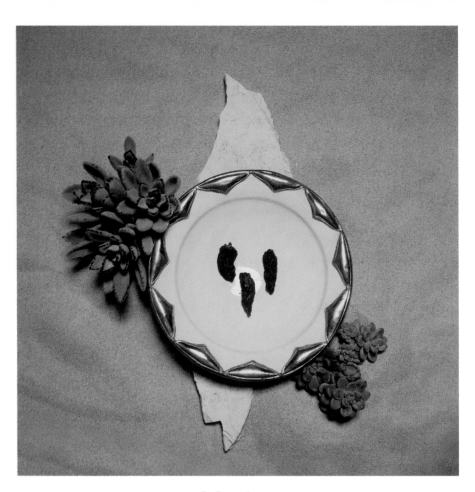

Morita

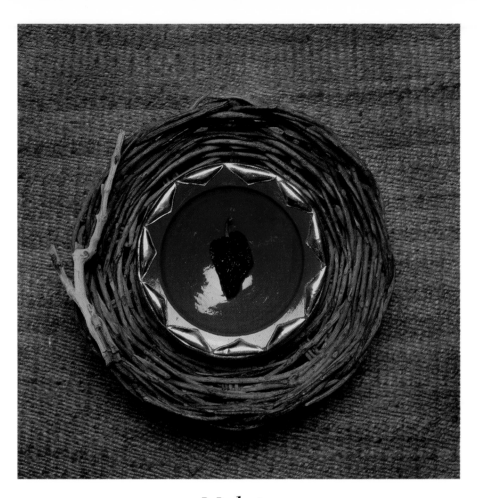

Mulato

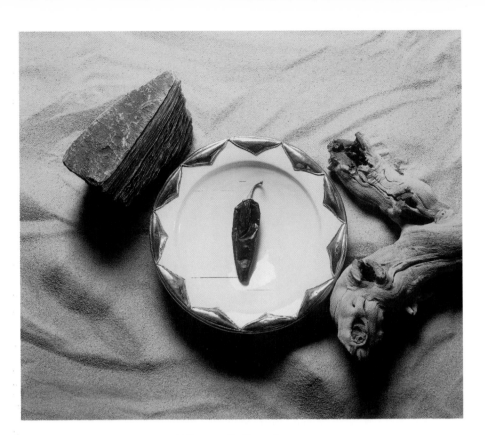

New Mexico

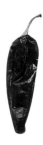

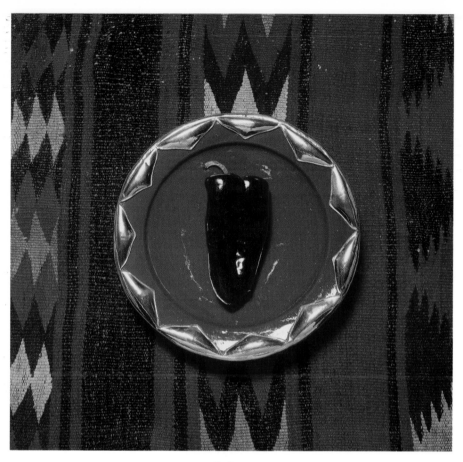

Poblano

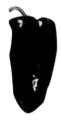

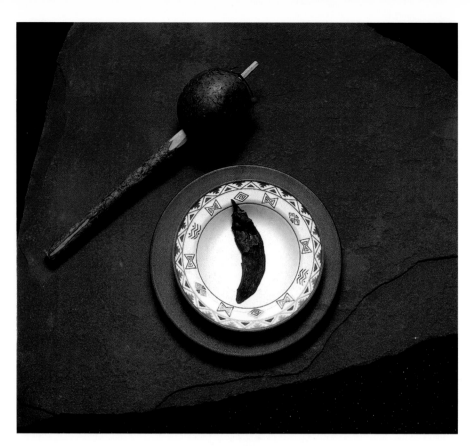

Pasado

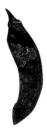

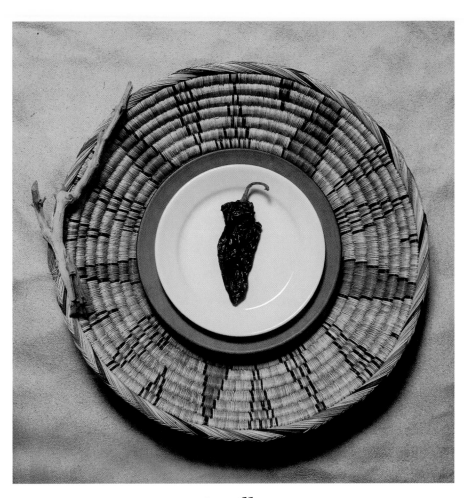

Pasilla

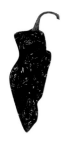

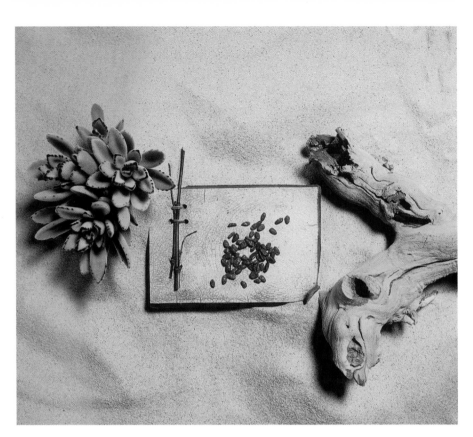

Pequin

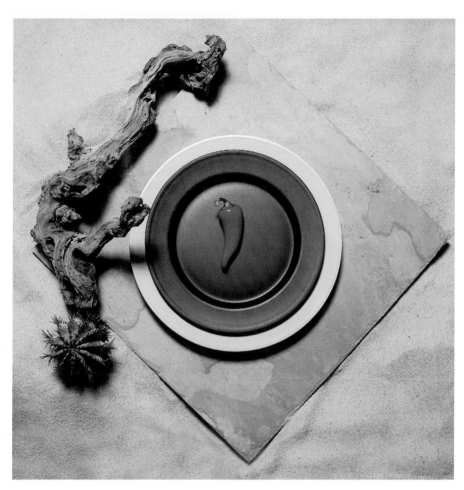

Red Jalapeno

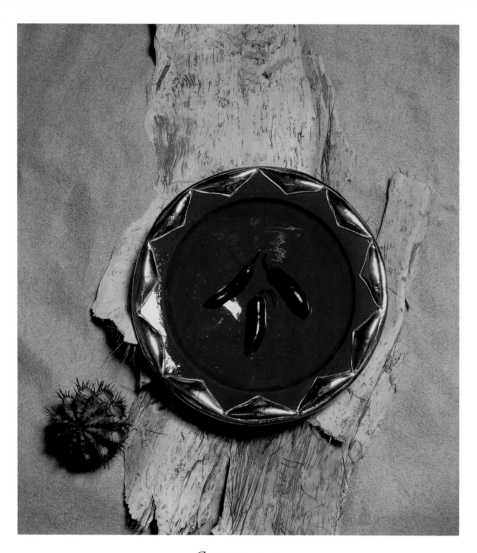

Serrano

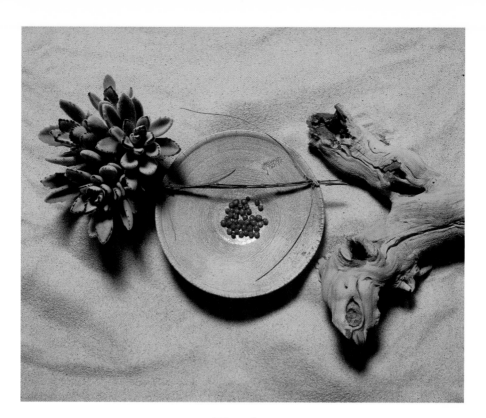

Tepin

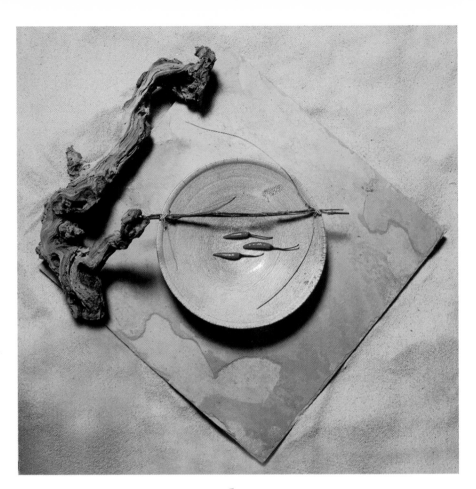

Thai

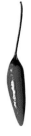

THE
CHILI PEPPER DIET

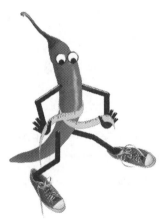

Now that we've had an education on increasing the flavor in our foods and a crash course on chilies themselves, let's look at the specifics of our diet. The focus of this program is eating foods that are good for you rather than eliminating those that are not. That means you'll be eating more health-enhancing fruits and vegetables, fish, whole grains and beans, and consuming less sugary, high-fat foods, chicken and red meat. Although lean red meat is allowed on this program, it should be limited to several times per month.

While many health experts recommend that you eat two servings of fish per week, this program doubles that amount to four servings per week. And there is a reason for this—not all proteins are created equal. Studies have shown that people who eat fish twice per week are less likely to suffer a fatal heart attack. Scientists credit their heart-healthy oils in preventing the development of a dangerous irregular heartbeat. Other studies have found that fish oil can lower high triglyceride levels—a common adverse side effect of low-fat diets. Moreover, a recent study conducted in Sweden found that the omega-3 fatty acids found in fish oil inhibit prostate cancer cell growth.

Another good reason to eat fish is that it seems to prevent depression. Exactly how fish achieves this remains unclear. Scientists speculate that eicosapentaenoic acid (EPA) and docsahexaenoic acid (DHA), two omega-3 fatty acids that are abundant in fatty fish like salmon, trout, mackerel and sardines, are responsible. Since over one-quarter of all women will struggle with depression in their lifetime, eating more fish seems very prudent advice.

Fish is not only good for your heart and mood, it can also help you lose weight. The fatty acids in fish seem to reduce cravings for high-carb foods. Moreover, the protein in fish is a great hunger-stopper. Fish is an excellent source of tyrosine, an amino acid that increases the production of the antihunger chemicals dopamine and norepinephrine. In one study, researchers found that overweight people who included a serving of fish every day in combination with a calorie-reduced diet lost 20 percent more weight than those who did not. It appears the protein in fish kept people from feeling hungry for longer periods of time than poultry or meat. That translates to eating fewer calories, and they lost weight.

HOW YOU WILL BE EATING

When it comes to losing weight, studies have shown that reducing the amount of calories you eat is still more important than exercise.

That's where chilies give you an edge—these pungent pods curb appetite. That translates to eating smaller portions of food without feeling hungry or deprived. Exercise enables you to shed pounds faster than with diet alone, and it is vital to maintaining your weight loss— it burns body fat and spares muscle tissue.

In the Chili Pepper Diet you will be eating five or six mini-meals per day. This style of eating, as opposed to the traditional three square meals per day, will help you burn calories at a more efficient rate. This becomes even more important as we age. It's important that you do not go below 1,200 calories per day, which can lower your metabolic rate. On this program, you should lose one to two pounds per week.

HOW THIS DIET WORKS

Calories do count! However, counting calories is about as much fun as balancing your checkbook. Most people won't do it. An easier way to control your calories is to count *serving sizes* instead of calories. The foundation of the Chili Pepper Diet is vegetables and fruits, as opposed to the traditional Food Pyramid, which focuses on grains. You'll eat at least eight to nine servings of fruits and vegetables per day, which is more than the Food Pyramid's recommended five servings of fruits and vegetables per day.

You can use the government's Food Pyramid as a guide if you want, but you will eat less than the recommended amounts of starches and fats. For instance, rather than eating six to eleven servings of starches, reduce that number to five if you're a women. If you're a man, increase your starches to six per day. Reserve alcohol and sweets for special treats.

GETTING STARTED

To trim your waistline, you need to trim your portion sizes. Two excellent tools will help you do this: keeping a food diary and using a kitchen scale. Keep a food diary for at least seven days; it will make you aware of both your eating patterns and portion sizes. I know it sounds like busy work, but it's not. Time and time again, this has proven to be one of the most effective tools you can use to lose weight. Without a food diary, researchers found that overweight women underestimated the amount of calories they ate by 500 calories per day, while that number jumps to 1,000 calories if they were obese.

Not only what you eat, but *when* you eat will pack on the pounds. I found that the majority of people in my study were eating just the opposite of how their bodies should be fed to manage their weight: They consumed the bulk of their calories after 6:00 P.M. A common eating pattern was skipping breakfast or lunch, snacking in the afternoon and eating a large dinner—which was followed by after-dinner noshing. In your twenties, you can get away with this funky eating pattern without getting fat. However, by the time you hit thirty-five, you can't.

Food Diary

	Sunday	Monday	Tuesday	Wednesday	Thursday	Friday	Saturday
Weight							
Exercise							
Mood							
Meals							
Breakfast							
Snack							
Lunch							
Snack							
Dinner							
Snack							

TIP: Record all the food you eat and how you are feeling when you eat. See if a pattern emerges.

EAT MORE OFTEN TO LOSE WEIGHT?

Eating a large quantity of food at one sitting encourages your body to store fat. This is especially true if you're a woman. Studies have found that women can't burn off more that 500 calories at any one given time. And those who eat a large meal at night (when the body is more efficient at storing fat, rather than burning fat) are sabotaging their weight-loss efforts. The body starts to decrease its metabolic rate as it prepares for sleep and does not burn calories as quickly as during the day. Researchers estimate that your metabolic rate drops by as much as 15 percent after the sun sets! Losing weight will be a lot easier if you choose an eating style that works *with* your natural biological rhythms, rather than fights them.

A SIMPLE WAY TO INCREASE YOUR METABOLISM

The body burns calories more efficiently when the food is eaten frequently and in smaller amounts. Scientists have found that eating five to six small meals per day increases metabolic rate above its basal level, which triggers the body to burn, rather than store fat. I know it sounds crazy, but eating actually increases your metabolic rate. Moreover, eating small amounts of food throughout the day doesn't stretch the stomach, so you'll feel full more quickly. Finally, there is evidence of improved cholesterol profiles and glucose tolerance among those who eat more frequently.

The trick to making this style of eating work is to keep your meals small. If you add two snacks to "regular-size" meals, you will gain weight. A general guideline is keeping your breakfast between 250 and 300 calories, while lunch and dinner should be in the range of 350 to 400 calories. Snacks should come in at 60 to 100 calories.

What Is Metabolism?

Metabolism is the sum of all chemical processes in the body that provide energy for the maintenance of life. It is often measured in calories per minute per kilogram body weight, which varies with your size and activity level. Basal metabolic rate (BMR) is the amount of calories your body needs to maintain basic body function, such as heartbeat, breathing, muscle tone, etc. Our BMR metabolism accounts for about 75 percent of the calories we expend per day.

After eating, your metabolism speeds up by 40 percent above the basal rate—a phenomenon known as "diet-induced thermic effect." Basically, it takes energy to break down food. Although this increase in metabolism doesn't compensate for the calories you take in, eating gives your metabolism a boost, which burns extra calories. If you eat at regular intervals, the thermic effect of food is responsible for about 5 to 10 percent of the calories you burn.

You can further enhance this increase in your metabolic rate by adding chilies to your mini-meals. Studies have shown that chilies increase this effect by a factor of twenty-five. In a study conducted at the Oxford Polytechnic Institute in England, researcher C. Henry and colleagues found that a mixture of chilies and hot mustard increased metabolic rate by 25 percent. You can maximize chilies' ability to increase metabolism and reduce appetite by combining a chili-spiked meal with a glass of green or black tea. In a study published in the *British Journal of Nutrition*, researchers found that combining caffeine and chilies had a synergistic effect.

Kitchen Tools

These items should be purchased before you start this diet. They will make it much easier to follow the program. Indispensable items are a food scale, nonstick pans, a coffee grinder, measuring spoons and a small hand chopper.

- **Kitchen scale:** Purchase the kind that you allows you to adjust the knob to zero. A terrific product is Cuisinart's Precision Portion Scale. I do not recommend digital kitchen food scales—they tend to break more often.
- **Measuring cups:** Two (liquid and dry).
- **Measuring spoons:** Two sets (plastic and metal).
- **Nonstick pans:** Eight-inch and ten-inch. It's not necessary to buy the most expensive brands—just replace them every four months.
- **Wooden utensils (large spoon, spatula):** Use with nonstick pans to prevent scratching the coating.
- **Kitchen scissors:** Use for slicing dry chilies.
- **Coffee grinder:** Use for grinding dry chilies only.
- **Zyliss cheese grinder:** Use for grinding Parmesan cheese.
- **Hand food choppers:** Use large for vegetables and onions; small for mincing fresh chilies.
- **Mandoline:** This tool will dramatically reduce your prep time in the kitchen slicing vegetables. Do not purchase expensive versions—plastic ones cost about twenty-six dollars and work just as well. The best plastic mandolines are from Japan, which allow you to adjust the thickness of the slice and offer several blades (fine-toothed and flat). If you have a Japanese market in your area, purchase a Benriner mandoline there.
- **Pressure cooker:** A wonderful tool for preparing soups, stews and beans. Cuts your time in the kitchen by half—the original "fast food" appliance.
- **Rice cooker:** Prepares perfectly cooked rice every time—both brown and white. Doubles as a steamer for veggies and fish.

- **Blender:** Use for preparing salsas, breadspreads and salad dressings.
- **Mortar and pestle:** The best tool for making fresh garlic pastes and roasted salsas. Choose a product that has a textured or rough surface (limestone, lava rock or textured ceramic), which creates tension to pulverize ingredients. Avoid products that have a slick interior, such as marble mortars.

PUTTING IT ALL TOGETHER

During the first week of the diet, you should weigh your foods so that you know what a proper serving size looks like. The most efficient way to measure fish, poultry, meat, cold cereals and cheese is with a food scale. Don't use measuring cups for these items—you won't get an accurate assessment. After several days, you'll be able to eyeball what a serving size looks like.

Other foods such as salad dressings, soups, sauces, rice and hot cereals and cooked pasta are best measured with measuring cups and spoons. If you are measuring a tablespoon of fruit spread or salad dressing, level off the spoon with a knife to get an accurate measurement. The easiest way to measure out two tablespoons of salad dressing is with a one-eighth cup measuring cup.

The portion sizes of juices, breakfast cereals and pasta are often misjudged.

- Do *not* pour cereal out of the box into your bowl. Weigh or measure your breakfast cereal *first*, then pour it into a bowl. A dense cereal, like Grape Nuts, packs 400 calories per cup, while bran flakes measure 120 calories per cup.
- If you drink orange juice, measure the juice into a serving cup *first*, then pour the juice into your juice glass. You'll be surprised at what a four-ounce serving size looks like—most people drink double or triple that amount. Designate one small glass as your "juice glass."
- Measure one cup of *cooked* pasta with a dry measuring cup. Eat pasta on a salad plate.

The Chili Pepper Diet Meal Plan

Women	Men
5 starch	6 starch
6 oz. protein	6 oz. protein
4 fruits	4 fruits
3–4+ vegetables	5–6 vegetables
1 cup nonfat milk	1 nonfat milk
3–5 chilies per day	3–5 chilies per day
Up to 23 grams of fat	20–28 grams of fat

MAINTENANCE

Once you have reached your goal weight, women should increase their fat grams to twenty-five to thirty grams of fats. Most women choose to add one tablespoon of regular salad dressing or one to two teaspoons of olive oil. Occasionally, you can indulge in a saturated fat—one tablespoon of cream cheese, a slice of cheese or a pat of butter. Also women should up their starches to six per day, and their chilies to five to eight per day. Men should increase their fat grams to thirty to thirty-five grams of fat per day, and up their starches to seven per day. Once a week, pick a meal where you can indulge by choosing one that is higher in fat than you would normally eat. Don't go overboard. For instance, if you are eating lobster, you might choose to dip every other bite in butter, alternating with a squeeze of fresh lemon juice. This technique works very well for me because I feel like I'm getting a little something extra. Also, you may enjoy an occasional glass of wine with your meal—just not more than one per week. Remember, it's important to weigh yourself several times per week. If you gain more than three pounds, it's time to get back on track.

Fat Exchanges

One serving: 35–40 calories; 3–5 grams of fat

1 tsp. olive or canola oil	5 large olives
	6–10 nuts
⅛ avocado	10 small olives
2 tsp. salad dressing	

One-Day Meal Plan

Breakfast

2 starch   1 cup oatmeal
1 nonfat dairy   with ½ cup nonfat milk
1 fruit   1¼ cups strawberries
water   coffee and water

Mid-morning snack

1 fruit   ¼ small cantaloupe with fresh lime juice
    and chili seasoning
water   water

Lunch

3 protein; 2 starch   Turkey (3 oz.) sandwich on whole wheat
½ vegetable   bread with extra tomatoes, lettuce
peppers   1–2 peppers (ancho; jalapeno)
1 vegetable   1 cup mixed green salad with 2 tablespoons
tea; water   Creamy Light Caesar Dressing (see recipe)
    or nonfat dressing
    Iced tea (unsweetened) and water

Mid-Afternoon snack

1 fruit   1 apple
water   water

Dinner

3 protein   3 oz. of grilled salmon
¼ vegetable   with ⅓ cup Cilantro Chutney (see recipe)
1 starch; ½ vegetable   ½ cup Rice Verde (see recipe)
½ vegetable   ½ cup steamed broccoli with Creamy Dill
peppers   Dressing (see recipe)
water   1 ancho (or pepper of choice)
    water

INDIVIDUALIZING THE MEAL PLAN

To lose weight, you do not need to follow all the recipes included in Part Three. In the study I did, lunches were often eaten in restaurants. Some people didn't cook. However, people did follow the rules of the diet: Eat five or six small meals per day, eat chilies several times per day, keep track of your fats (in general, women should not exceed 23 grams of fat per day, while men should limit fats to 28 grams per day), limit your portion sizes of starches and protein, eat four fruits and four vegetables per day and one serving of nonfat dairy product. Also, you'll need to take a calcium supplement (1,000 mg per day); drink eight to ten eight-ounce-glasses of water per day; walk for thirty to forty-five minutes, three to four times per week; drink one serving of black or green tea each day; and eat dinner between 5:30 and 7:00 P.M.

Some people preferred to front-load their starches during the day. These tended to be "morning people." Night owls did better adding a small serving of protein to their breakfast—either a hard-boiled egg or a one-ounce serving of smoked salmon with their toasted bagel. Some people wanted a larger portion of fish (four ounces *cooked*) at dinner, and reduced the amount of turkey or fat-free ham on their sandwich to two ounces at lunch. Sometimes a fruit was skipped mid-morning and two were eaten in the afternoon. It's important that you find a style of eating that works for you.

The people who got the best results added chilies to at least three meals per day: breakfast, lunch, mid-afternoon snack and dinner. Basically, this worked out to chilies being consumed at three- to four-hour intervals. However, some people balked at eating chilies at breakfast. Since overweight people tend to overeat in the afternoon and evening, I advised to add chilies to lunch, mid-afternoon snack and dinner to cover these high-risk eating periods.

BREAKFAST

Many people on the Chili Pepper Diet ate the same breakfast nearly every weekday, and that's fine. It seemed that simplicity, not variety, is what most people wanted on a busy workday morning. If that sounds familiar, reserve recipes that require cooking beyond hitting a microwave button for the weekend.

My advice is to choose a breakfast plan that fits your lifestyle. What's most important is that you do *not* skip this meal. Even if you're not a morning person, it's *crucial* that you get into the habit of eating breakfast. It will get your metabolism up and running, and prevent a binge at lunch.

Keep your breakfast low-fat and filling. For instance, if you choose to eat cereal, pair it with a serving of nonfat milk and a fresh fruit. It's important that you use nonfat milk for two very good reasons: not only does cutting the fat slash calories, it appears to reduce appetite. According to Barbara Rolls, professor of nutrition at Pennsylvania State University, drinking milk with your meal makes you full sooner, which helps you eat less. And the lighter the milk, the more it curbs your appetite. Also make breads more filling by adding a small serving of protein and vegetables. Think of every meal as an opportunity to include vegetables.

In the beginning of the study I conducted, many people resisted eating chilies at breakfast. Eating spicy food after rolling out of bed didn't sound appealing. However, as they got accustomed to the diet, something interesting occurred: Chilies started to be incorporated into morning meals. And for a very good reason—chilies not only curbed the dieters' appetites, but made them feel "more alive."

In many ways, eating chilies is similar to drinking coffee. Most people don't like coffee the first time they try it; it tastes bitter. However, they do like the way it makes them feel, and so they continue to drink it. Soon, its acrid flavor is no longer an issue. In time, just the smell of a fresh pot of brewing coffee lures people out of their warm, comfortable beds.

BAGELS ARE NOT DIETARY PARIAHS

Although some diets advocate that you avoid bagels, this program does not. More than half of the people in the study made bagels a regular morning meal—and they lost weight! The trick to making bagels work is reduce your portion size—eat one half of a large deli bagel or one small (two-and-a-half- to three-ounce) bagel. Also, include a small serving of protein and a side of tomatoes and peppers with your meal. For instance, pair your bagel with one ounce of smoked salmon (or one whole poached or hard-boiled egg) and four slices of tomato and minced jalapenos. If jalapenos are too hot, eat an ancho before your meal.

BAGEL BITES

Bagels seem to be getting bigger every year. According to the U.S.D.A. Handbook for food exchanges, half a bagel is the equivalent of one starch. However, that serving size is based on a two-ounce (fifty-seven-gram) bagel—and that size bagel no longer exists! Over the last five years, a standard bagel has increased from two ounces to four ounces. Although most people would balk at eating four slices of whole wheat toast for breakfast, they think nothing of downing its caloric equivalent by eating a four-ounce bagel. Your best bet is to weigh bagels—some delis serve 6.2 ounce bagels!

If you're having breakfast at a deli, order a mini-bagel and count it as two starch, or eat half a regular-sized 4-ounce bagel and count it as two starch. If you're buying a supermarket bagel, choose the brand that is smallest in size.

LUNCH AND DINNER

Generally, lunches and dinners are interchangeable. You should try to get between 350 and 400 calories per meal, and at least twenty grams of protein. For instance, if you're eating a frozen low-fat vegetarian meal that supplies only ten grams of protein, make up the difference with a glass of nonfat milk or a serving of nonfat yogurt. Also, these meals should include several whole chilies, a serving of fruit and two servings of vegetables. If your entree does not include chilies, eat a whole chili before the meal, or add chilies to your salad, soup or sandwich. It's recommended that you eat the majority of your starches during the day (at breakfast and lunch), and limit starches to a small serving (no more than two) at your evening meal. For instance, don't consume a large serving of pasta (2 cups) at dinner. Limit your portion to 1 cup.

SNACKS

Snacking is a key part of this diet—it keeps your metabolism revved in high gear and prevents binges. While most of us grab carbohydrate-heavy chips or pretzels, these tasty morsels are far from being the ideal snack. A much better choice is fruit.

The fiber in fruit keeps hunger at bay for longer periods of time because it's more filling; it slows down the release of glucose into the bloodstream and provides a steady source of energy. Also, choosing fruit for your snacks is an easy way to ensure you get your four fruits per day.

I found that people avoid fruits because they lack flavor. And they have a valid point—most conventionally grown fruit tastes like water. Buy organically grown fruit instead—they really do taste better. This is especially true with apples, which should be one of your four fruits per day. Also, you can enhance the flavor of fruits by adding fresh lime juice and chili seasoning (Chef Merito's Salt Lemon and Chili seasoning or fresh lime juice with Chef Merito's Pikos Picosos). This seasoning technique works with melons (cantaloupe, watermelon and honeydew) and apples.

Eat a variety of fruits to get the full range of this food group's health-promoting benefits and phytochemicals. The fruits that seem to put the biggest dent in appetite are apples and berries. A great morning fruit is berries. Apples are a good choice for counteracting the mid-afternoon energy slump. Eat two apples or add a serving of low-fat cheese or nonfat yogurt if you feel especially hungry. Tropical fruits are a wonderful substitute for rich desserts. Don't make the mistake of eating only bananas and oranges—you'll get bored. Every so often, try a different afternoon snack. A good alternative choice is air-popped popcorn, sprinkled with chili seasoning.

WHAT IS A SERVING SIZE?

The amount of food you eat at a meal may be more than one serving. For instance, a one-cup dinner portion of spaghetti will count as two servings of starch. A portion of fish, poultry or meat will be three ounces, cooked. One supermarket (three-ounce) bagel will count as three starches, while one cup of Raisin Bran or oatmeal counts as two starches.

Food Exchanges

STARCH/BREAD/GRAIN

One serving: 60–100 calories (average 80 calories)
2–3 gm protein; 0 gm fat; 15 gm carbohydrate

Cereals

1 oz. Grape Nuts
1 oz. Shredded Wheat
½ cup of hot cereal (oatmeal, Wheatena, Cream of Wheat)
½ cup Raisin Bran

Breads

½ pita bread
½ English muffin
½ 2-ounce bagel
1 6-inch corn tortilla

1 low-fat 8-inch flour tortilla
1 slice of whole wheat bread (1 oz.)
2 rice cakes (4-inch)
4–6 crackers (whole wheat; low-fat)

Grains

½ cup rice, brown or white, cooked
½ cup barley, cooked

3 cups air-popped popcorn

Starchy vegetables

½ cup sweet potato, yam
½ cup potato

½ medium baked potato (3 oz.)
½ cup corn, peas, winter squash

FRUIT

One serving: 60–100 calories; 0–1 gm protein; 15–25 gm carb
One medium fresh fruit

apple
orange
pear
persimmon
peach
½ cup chopped fresh fruit
½ cup of orange juice
½ banana (9-inch)
1 cup berries

½ mango
½ papaya
¾ cup of pineapple
½ grapefruit
15 green seedless grapes
½ cantaloupe; 1 cup melon balls
2 apricots, plums, figs or kiwis
1 oz. dried fruit

VEGETABLES

One serving: 25 calories; 2 gm protein; 0 gm fat; 5 gm carb
½ cup of cooked or 1 cup raw vegetables
1 cup of raw leafy greens
⅓ roasted salsa
½ cup chopped salsa

artichokes
beans (green, wax, Italian)
bok choy
broccoli
brussels sprouts
cabbage
carrots
cauliflower
greens (collard, mustard, turnip)
kale
kohlrabi

leeks
mushrooms
okra
onions
peapods
bell peppers
rutabaga
spinach
summer squash, crookneck squash
tomato
zucchini

PROTEIN

One lunch or dinner portion: 3–4 ounces, cooked; average = 150–200 calories
1 oz. = 35–100 calories (average 50 calories)

One Ounce	Protein	Fat	Carb
Lean	7 gm	1–3 gm	0 gm
Medium fat	7 gm	5 gm	0 gm
High fat	7 gm	8 gm	0 gm

1 oz. chicken breast, skinless
1 oz. turkey breast, skinless
¼ cup albacore tuna, packed in water
1 oz. all fresh and frozen fish (salmon, tuna, trout, lox, Chilean sea bass, anchovies)
1 oz. shrimp, clams, lobster

1 cup nonfat milk
3 egg whites
1 whole egg (up to 4 whole eggs per week)
½ cup beans, cooked

Lean Meats (limit to several times per month)

1 oz. top round, cooked
1 oz. filet mignon, cooked
1 oz. eye of round, cooked
1 oz. flank steak, cooked

1 oz. sirloin tip, cooked
1 oz. (5 to 7 percent fat) hamburger

NUTRITION 101

The majority of your carbohydrates should be whole grains, fruits, vegetables and legumes, which are a lot healthier than refined carbohydrates. Complex carbs not only have less calories, but supply more vitamins, minerals and phytochemicals. They also contain more fiber, which tames your hunger. Fiber-rich foods stay in your stomach longer, which delays the time you'll feel hungry again. Moreover, fiber slows down the absorption of glucose. Finally, if you're trying to reduce your cholesterol, soluble fiber (the type found in oats, beans, vegetables and fruits) can lower LDL cholesterol (the bad kind), which reduces your risk for heart disease.

If you eat a refined carbohydrate (pasta, bagel or pita bread), pair it with a serving of protein, lots of vegetables or a small amount of fat to slow down the absorption of glucose. For instance, order a pasta dish with a low-fat marinara sauce and seafood. Also, be sure to include chilies with the meal!

Proteins

Protein is found in meats, fish, poultry, cheese, eggs and peanut butter. Milk, yogurt and beans also contain a fair amount of protein. Protein builds muscle and facilitates certain enzyme reactions in the body. If your body doesn't get enough protein, it will start to break down its own muscle for protein, which leaves you with less lean muscle mass. You want to avoid this situation when you're trying to lose weight since it will lower your metabolic rate.

To get the best results on this program, you should eat six ounces of protein each day. After capsaicin is activated by metabolites in the liver, it attaches to protein and is transported to various sites in the body. In animal studies, researchers found that low-protein diets actually impaired the ability of capsaicin to reduce high cholesterol levels.

FATS

For the last decade, nutritionists have been telling us to reduce the amount of fat in our diet. However, that advice may have only been partly correct. As the results of studies emerge, it's becoming increasingly clear that we need to limit certain fats while increasing others.

There are several types of fats, and some fats are better than others. Healthy fats prevent premature aging by supplying your body with essential fatty acids and fat-soluble vitamins, which are necessary for making hormones and maintaining cell structures. They also make you feel more satisfied. The fats you should limit are saturated fats. Avoid partially hydrogenated fats, which can wreak havoc with your body.

Saturated fats—completely saturated with hydrogen—are solid at room temperature and are found in animal products and tropical oils. Saturated fats raise total cholesterol and LDL cholesterol, which increases your risk for heart disease. Foods high in saturated fats include: whole-fat dairy products, butter, cheese, egg yolks, fatty meats, poultry skin, dark poultry meat, lard and tropical oils (palm, palm kernel and coconut). However, many junk foods are also loaded with saturated fats—crackers, snack foods, cookies and pastries are often made with tropical oil.

The most hazardous fats appear to be partially hydrogenated oils, or trans-fats. These artificially manufactured fats are created by injecting hydrogen into polyunsaturated oils, which makes them more solid. Trans-fats increase your risk of heart disease by raising LDL cholesterol and lowering HDL cholesterol. Some researchers feel that trans-fats unfavorably affect the enzymes used for fat

Food Shopping Guide

Cereals and Grains	Fish	Frozen Foods	Bread	Dairy
Nutrigrain	Lox	Low-fat frozen meals	Whole wheat bread	Nonfat milk
Shredded Wheat	Salmon			Light sour cream
		Pre-cooked frozen shrimp	Corn tortillas	
	Tuna			Nonfat cream cheese
Multigrain			Bagels (2.5- to 3-oz., plain)	
	Chilean Sea bass	Frozen stir-fry vegetable medleys		Lifetime Nonfat Mozzarella Shredded Cheese
Wheatena			Low-fat flour tortillas (8-inch)	
Roman Meal	Trout			
		Frozen veggie burgers		
Raisin Bran	Swordfish		Pita bread	Kraft 2% Milk Fat Cheese (slices only)
Cream of Wheat	Scallops	Frozen broccoli		
Oatmeal				
				Friendship Spreadable (1% Milkfat)
White rice				
				Whipped Low-Fat Cottage Cheese
Brown rice				
Barley				
				Parmesan cheese
Lentils				
				Nonfat plain yogurt

Canned Foods	Produce	Meat	Other
Starkist Albacore Tuna, packed in water (3-oz. cans)	Berries (strawberries, blueberries)	Prepackaged fat-free chicken, turkey and ham slices	Low-fat marinara sauce
Progresso Lentil Soup, Hearty Black Bean Soup, Chicken and Wild Rice Soup	Pre-cut vegetables: baby carrots, broccoli	Precooked roasted chicken (breast only, remove skin)	Classico Tomato & Basil Pasta Sauce
	Bag salad	5–7% fat hamburger	Tryson House All Natural Flavor Sprays: Buttery Delight, Mesquite Mist, Italian Mist
Canned beans: garbanzo, kidney, pinto, black	Apples	Lean meats	
	Tomatoes	Eggs	Imagine Natural Organic Free Range Chicken Broth
Rosarita Low-Fat Refried Black Beans	Potatoes		
	Celery		Swanson 99% Fat-Free Chicken Broth
Chipotle chilies in adobo sauce	Chives		
	Cantaloupe		Imagine Creamy Tomato Soup
	Papaya		
	Peaches		Olive oil
	Limes		Japanese seasoned rice wine vinegar
	Bananas		
	Orange juice		Low-fat & nonfat salad dressings
	Fresh & dried chilies		Nonfat mayo
	Prepared salsas		Dijon mustard
			Puréed ginger & garlic in a jar

metabolism, and alter the number and size of fat cells. Moreover, trans-fats deplete omega-3 fatty acids (the good-for-your-heart oils), and decrease the insulin response, which is undesirable for diabetics.

Furthermore, when you heat and reheat partially hydrogenated oils (a common practice in fast-food restaurants), trans-fats create dangerous free radicals. These fats are rampant in stick margarine, fried foods, fast foods and almost every packaged food you can imagine.

There are several types of unsaturated fats. Polyunsaturated fats, found in corn, soybean, safflower and sunflower oils, should be eaten in moderation. While polyunsaturated fats can lower LDL cholesterol, a diet high in polyunsaturated fats increases triglyceride levels and decreases HDL cholesterol. Moreover, these poly oils are the most likely to form DNA-damaging free radicals when heated, which have been linked to cancer.

Foods that contain healthy fats are key players in the Chili Pepper Diet. Mono fats and omega-3s can decrease your risk for a heart attack or stroke. These healthy fats support brain function and hormone production. Moreover, these oils are good for your heart—they can lower total cholesterol, triglycerides and LDL cholesterol, while increasing HDL cholesterol levels. Omega-3s are found in most varieties of fish, and they are especially abundant in fatty fish. Numerous studies have shown that people who eat six to eight ounces of fish per week experience significantly fewer heart attacks and strokes.

Monounsaturated fats are derived from plants and are found in olive, peanut and canola oil, avocados, almonds, cashews and peanuts. Monounsaturated fats lower the risk of heart disease by slightly lowering LDL cholesterol, while slightly increasing HDL cholesterol.

The goal in the Chili Pepper Diet is to substitute as many healthy fats as you can for saturated fats and partially hydrogenated oils. However, don't load up on avocados and olive oil since eating too many healthy fats has a point of diminishing return—they are still fats and will pack on the pounds. Make substitutions—eat more fish; cook with nonstick flavor sprays, use breadspreads instead of mayonnaise; use small amounts of olive oil to flavor food (instead of cooking with it); use nonfat dairy products and add small amounts of cheese as a condiment. Don't completely eliminate red meat from your diet—select lean cuts of meat, and eat smaller portions on an occasional basis.

Calcium

Dairy products are often the first foods to go when you're trying to lose weight. And for good reason—many dairy products are high in fat. However, calcium just might be one of your best lines of defense in the fight against fat.

In a recent study published in the *Journal of Clinical Endocrinology and Metabolism*, researchers found that a low-calcium diet promotes your body to secrete hormones that lower your metabolic rate. In another study involving hypertensive African Americans, researchers found that increasing calcium levels with supplements resulted in significant weight loss. These researchers uncovered that low calcium levels prompt the body to release hormones that switch fat cells from a fat-burning to a fat-storing mode.

Rather than dropping dairy from your diet, select mainly nonfat dairy products. You can also add nonfat skim milk powder to cooked breakfast cereals, soups, sauces, mashed potatoes or skim milk to up their calcium content, protein and flavor.

Dairy products are not the only way to get more calcium into your menu plan. Vegetables, such as collard greens, bok choy, kale, hijiki, and fish with edible bones (canned salmon), are other excellent sources. However, the caveat with eating leafy greens for calcium is you need to eat large servings. For instance, you need to eat two one-cup servings of cooked collard greens to get the same amount of calcium that one serving of skim milk provides.

Calcium Supplements

On the Chili Pepper Diet, it is recommended to shoot for 1,300 to 1,500 milligrams of calcium per day. While one to two servings of nonfat dairy products per day will get you closer to that goal, you will still come up short. Make up the difference with supplements.

Many types of calcium supplements are available. Avoid calcium supplements that use bone meal or dolomite as the calcium source—many brands contain lead. Calcium citrate (Citracal) has the advantage of being the most readily absorbed form. Antacids, such as Tums EX, are made from calcium carbonate—chalk. They are one of the least expensive supplements you can buy and have the added advantage of coming in a variety of tasty flavors, which makes it easier to chew them between meals.

To boost the absorption of calcium, either take it on an empty stomach (before you go to bed) or with foods that contain vitamin C (citrus). Dairy products also enhance its absorption. Avoid taking calcium supplements with high-fiber foods or caffeinated beverages, such as coffee, soda or tea, which may impair calcium's absorption.

The best way to take calcium is to divide up the doses throughout the day, rather than taking one large dose. The body can only absorb just so much calcium at one time and will excrete the rest. For instance, if you are going for 1,000 milligrams of supplemental calcium per day, take 500 milligrams in the morning and 500 milligrams in the evening. Don't exceed 2,000 milligrams of calcium per day, which is linked to an increased risk of developing kidney stones.

Many over-the-counter calcium supplements contain lead. Below are a few of the popular brands that were tested, with the micrograms of lead given per 1,500 mg of calcium.

Product	Lead
Caltrate 600	3.43
Calcium 600 mg	3.18
Liqui-Cal Calcium 600 softgels	2.95
Oscal 500	1.74
Oyster Shell Calcium, 500 mg with vitamin D	1.95
Pharmaceutical Grade Calcium 600	No lead
Renagel	No lead
Calci-Chew	No lead
Tums EX	No lead
TUMS Ultra	Contains lead

Source: "Alert on Lead in Calcium," *Los Angeles Times* (Oct. 2, 2000), Health Section, from the Associated Press

Water

Studies have shown that many times when you think you're hungry, you're actually thirsty. And dehydration can be a major contributor of fatigue. Many times when you're tired and crave sugary snacks as a pick-me-up, what your body really needs is a glass of water.

There are many types of water to choose from: tap, mineral, distilled, spring and purified. If your tap water smells or tastes of chlorine, avoid it. Chlorine is a potent oxidizing agent that has been linked to arteriosclerosis. Moreover, some tap water contains toxic materials, such as lead, pesticides, fertilizers or radioactive agents.

Unfortunately, bottled spring and mineral water may not be a better choice. In 1999, the Natural Resources Defense Council reported that 23 of the 103 brands of bottled water violated California's limits for contaminants. They contained unsafe levels of bacteria, arsenic and carcinogenic chemicals.

I struggled to drink sixty-four ounces of water per day until I discovered distilled water. Not only is distilled water the purest water, it also has a much smoother taste compared to other types of bottled water because the minerals have been removed—it just went down easier. Many people in my study who had trouble drinking enough water preferred distilled water once they tried it.

The best way to incorporate more water into your diet is to set a schedule—drink two glasses with every meal (including snacks). Also, keep a bottle of water in your car, and another near your desk at work.

Alcohol

It's not news to anyone that alcohol will pack on the pounds by adding extra calories. However that's only half the story. In a study investigating the effects of alcohol on metabolism, researchers found that alcohol causes the body to burn fat at a much slower rate than usual, which makes it harder to lose weight. In a study published in *The New England Journal of Medicine*, Dr. Paolo Suter and his colleagues found that three ounces of alcohol suppresses fat metabolism, and reduced the body's ability to burn fat by almost one-third.

Another good reason to limit alcohol when you're trying to lose weight is that it impairs sleep. And there appears to be a big connection with getting a bad night's sleep and being fat. While alcohol initially acts a sedative, there's a rebound arousal effect later in the night. Although it helps you fall asleep, you won't stay asleep. And if you do manage to make it through the night, you won't feel rested in the morning. To feel rejuvenated, the body needs to experience a stage of sleep known as Slow Wave Sleep (deep sleep), which alcohol disrupts.

Being sleep-deprived makes us feel sluggish and moody. It makes it harder for us to concentrate, short-circuits our memory and renders us less able to handle stress. However, a bad night's sleep does more damage than just make us feel bad—it also makes us eat more food and make less muscle. The body interprets a lack of sleep as stress and responds by producing more cortisol. Elevated cortisol levels not only increase our appetite (especially for carbs and fatty foods), they also deplete our muscles by promoting cellular breakdown.

In my study, we recommended limiting alcohol intake to three ounces of wine at a time and restricting it to special occasions.

This appears to be very prudent advice. In a recent study conducted by Dr. Kahn et al., researchers found that women who drank liquor or beer one to four times per week were more likely to gain abdominal fat. However, wine did not increase their waistline and appears to be a better choice.

Chilies

Build up a tolerance to chilies slowly to minimize the possibility of gastrointestinal upset.

- If you are new to chilies, start with two ancho chilies per day (lunch and dinner).
- Eat the serving of food that contains chilies first, such as salad with pickled peppers, baked potato with salsa or fish sauced with salsa. If your meal does not contain chilies, chomp on a chili before you eat your meal.
- Chilies reduce appetite best if the meal is low-fat and includes a serving of protein.
- When possible, combine chilies with garlic, onions and ginger in dishes. Capsaicin increases circulation, and enhances the

healing powers of these herbs (onions have been shown to be beneficial in diabetes).

- Avoid hot sauces that contain oleoresin capsaicin, such as the brands Insanity, Suicide and Death. These incendiary sauces can cause blistering, shortness of breath and spontaneous vomiting. I experienced nausea and a ringing in my ears—it was not a pleasant experience. Moreover, these products do nothing to enhance the flavor of food—they're just hot. Why bother?

- Do not eat a chili-spiked meal within two hours of bedtime. Chilies increase body temperature and metabolic rate, which may interfere with getting a restful sleep.

- Make an effort to eat dinner between 5:30 P.M. and 7:00 P.M. Your body does not burn calories as efficiently after that.

Precautions

- This program is not recommended for people who suffer from kidney disease, peptic ulcers, hiatal hernias, gastritis or inflammatory bowel conditions. Consult your physician before starting this program.

- If you have diabetes, consult a registered dietitian or physician before starting this program.

- Several studies have found that asthmatics are more sensitive to capsaicin, and that inhaling chili powder can trigger an asthmatic attack. Other studies have found that eating chilies actually prevented asthmatic attacks. If you suffer from asthma, consult your physician before starting this program.

- Some brands of pickled chilies contain sulfites. If you are allergic to sulfites, be sure to read labels before eating any pickled chili. Also, ask the manager at a restaurant if the chilies at the salad bar contain this preservative.

- A recent study found that chilies decrease the absorption of aspirin.

CHILI PEPPERS 101

There are many ways you can incorporate chilies into your diet. Toss pickled chilies in salad or on a sandwich. "Salsa" your foods, rather than sauce your foods. Sprinkle chili powder into soups, or simply munch on a chili before a meal.

If you've never eaten chilies, start slowly. Start with chilies that are listed as having 1,000 Scoville heat units. In the dieters I studied, many people started with two to three ancho chilies per day—one at lunch and one at dinner. A few people also ate this chili with their mid-afternoon snack if they felt hungry. This is a terrific pod to introduce your palate to chilies; it has a rich, sweet flavor that is reminiscent of a raisin. This mild chili works best at reducing your appetite when eaten alone (like a serving of fruit) and at the beginning of your meal. When you eat it, you will feel a tickling sensation on your tongue.

To enjoy an ancho, remove its stem, split it open from top to bottom and then shake out the seeds. Then roll up the ancho chili like a cigarette, and cut it with kitchen shears into thin strips. You can add the ancho strips to low-fat food, or simply eat them.

Even these mild chilies were a bit hot for one person. He started with four pepperoncini peppers and several canned green chilies per day. The pepperoncini chili is a very mild pickled pepper that works well tossed into a salad. However, you'll get better results if you eat this chili alone at the beginning of your meal (do not remove the seeds). If you aren't sensitive to the heat of a chili, don't choose this pod, since it's far too mild.

As you build up a tolerance for chilies, move up the Scoville scale to the hotter varieties. Add pickled jalapenos to your sandwiches and salsas. If these chilies are a bit hot, remove the seeds. As you build up a tolerance, increase the amount of chilies, and do not remove the seeds. If you start to feel hungry between meals, now is the time to double the amount of chilies you are eating, or use hotter chilies. For instance, if you were using jalapeno chilies, try serrano chilies or de àrbols.

Work your way up to at least five chilies per day and eat them at regular intervals. Top your breakfast eggs with a spicy salsa, toss chopped chilies into a salad at lunch and sprinkle ground arbols into your bean soup at dinner. Be creative!

There appears to be a threshold with these fiery fruits. Eventually, people found a level of chilies that consistently worked for reducing their appetite, and they remained at that level. The number and type of chilies varied from person to person. Some people ate more than eight chilies per day, while other found five chilies did the trick. The magic number seemed to be around five to six whole chilies per day, spaced at three-hour intervals.

The Best Way to Increase Your Tolerance to Chilies

The burning sensation produced by a chili is caused by capsaicin, which irritates trigeminal nerves (pain receptors located in the mouth, nose and stomach). When these sensory nerves are irritated by capsaicin, they release substance P, a chemical messenger that sends pain signals to the brain. However, eating chilies on a regular basis confuses the substance P receptors, which explains why you build up a tolerance to capsaicin. If you eat chilies several times a day, you will soon build up a tolerance to their heat. A good way to increase your tolerance to capsaicin is by eating salsa. These vegetable-based sauces are the perfect vehicle for delivering increasing amounts of chilies.

In many ways, there are similarities in how nicotine and capsaicin work in the body. For instance, a person will start smoking a few cigarettes per day, and eventually work his or her way to a pack a day and stay at that level. Unless that person is under stress, he or she continues to smoke the same number of cigarettes per day. The same phenomenon seemed to hold true for chilies.

In my study, some quickly ascended to eating serranos, while others didn't make it past anchos. An interesting observation was individuals who were extroverted or creative appeared to have a greater capacity for eating spicy foods. According to Dr. Alan Hirsch, neurological director of the Smell and Taste Research Foundation in Chicago, people who are risk-takers, such as firefighters, have a preference for spicy foods. These people inherently have lower levels of serotonin and choose foods, hobbies or professions that raise levels of adrenaline, which makes them feel more "alive."

- Start with two whole chilies per day. Ancho chilies are an excellent choice if you're new to chilies. If you are used to eating chilies, start with one jalapeno chili per meal.
- Eat chilies at regular intervals to decrease your appetite. If you're new to chilies, start by adding chilies to your lunch and dinner. Then add chilies to your morning meal and snacks as you become accustomed to the heat.
- Increase your tolerance to chilies with salsas. Start slowly (remove seeds) and gradually increase the amount of and intensity of chili.
- If you use crushed red pepper flakes, start with one-quarter teaspoon per meal.
- Men tend to like chilies that have a smoky flavor, while women tend to go for the fruity-flavored pods.
- If you have high blood pressure, use dried chilies. Sun-dried

chilies have significantly higher amounts of potassium, which has been shown to reduce increases in blood pressure associated with high salt intake. Avoid canned chilies—the canning process leeches potassium. Also limit pickled chilies.

Chili Equivalents

- One tablespoon of chili paste is equivalent to two chilies.
- One teaspoon of hot chili powder is equivalent to four chilies.

How to Incorporate Chilies If You Don't Like Spicy Food

- Use mild chilies and up the amount. For instance, eat five pepperoncini peppers and two canned green chilies instead of one ancho. While the best health benefits come from fresh chilies, canned chilies are a viable option for people who are *very* sensitive to the heat of chilies. They're also easy to use and convenient. So, for people who need to slowly acclimate their palate to chilies, or those who don't have a lot of time for food preparation, canned green chilies make a great "starter chili." However, fresh chilies have more health benefits and a better taste than canned overall.
- Eat chilies with a dairy product. One study participant topped her bagel with nonfat cream cheese, canned green chilies and tomatoes to introduce her palate to chilies.

Why Are Some People More Sensitive to Chilies?

In Mexico, the more hot chilies a man can eat, the more "macho" or masculine he is. However, tolerating the heat of a chili has more to do with your genes (and anatomy) than testosterone levels—it's determined by the amount of taste buds and trigeminal nerves (pain receptors) on your tongue. It's also determined by your medical history!

Yet, there is some truth backing this "macho" idea, but it's not for the reason these cultures presume—women are more likely than men to be super-tasters. Approximately 50 percent of the population are medium-tasters, which means that they have an average amount of taste buds per centimeter on their tongue. The remaining population is divided into super-tasters, who have more taste buds, and nontasters, who have very few. Super-tasters are nearly twice as sensitive to the bite of a chili as nontasters.

Also, studies have found that people who have a history of suffering from earaches (*otitis media*) can have either more or less taste buds. People who have suffered a head injury will have less and be less sensitive to the burning effect of capsaicin.

Super-tasters and medium-tasters are also more sensitive to sweet, bitter and fatty tastes. In a study conducted at Rutgers University, researchers found that medium-tasters and super-tasters could differentiate between fat levels in salad dressings (40 percent fat vs. 10 percent fat), while nontasters could not. Also, only the nontasters preferred the taste of the oilier salad dressing. These researchers speculate that the same receptors that distinguish taste also perceive textures and fat. Perhaps this explains why people who like chilies also tend to like fatty foods—they need more stimulation to perceive the same sensations that "normal" people do.

Putting Out the Burn

Folk remedies for putting out a chili burn include beer, tequila, bread, sugar, water, citrus fruits, beans, carbonated drinks and dairy products. It's presumed these items work by either diluting, or absorbing, capsaicin. Unfortunately, the majority of these rescue remedies don't work. The problem is that capsaicin tightly binds to nerve receptor sites in the mouth, and it is difficult to pry loose.

The most effective antidote for a chili burn is cold milk. Researchers have found that the protein in milk, casein, strips the capsaicin from the nerve receptor sites in the taste buds. Basically, the casein acts like a soap and lifts the capsaicin from the nerve.

I found the most effective way to use milk is to take a large gulp, then tilt your head toward the floor, which pools the milk toward the front of the tongue. Hold the milk in your mouth (do not swallow) for at least one to two minutes, then rinse vigorously. Repeat this procedure at least two more times. Have another dose of milk handy— your mouth will still be on fire when you spit out the milk. However, you should feel no pain while milk is in your mouth. In takes about eight minutes to put out the fire.

Tip: Cloves intensify the burning effect of chilies. In Mexico, ground cloves are a "secret ingredient" in certain regional salsas. Reduce the amount of chilies, or heat level of a chili, if you add cloves to a salsa.

Supplements to Take While on the Chili Pepper Diet

While on this diet and, in fact, for good health overall, take the following supplements.

- Take a complete multivitamin and mineral supplement that contains 100 percent of the daily requirements for most nutrients.
- Supplement with 1,000 milligrams of calcium. A good product

is Citracal, which is lead-free and contains vitamin D (enhances calcium absorption). Since only 500 milligrams of calcium can be absorbed at one time, divide the dose (500 milligrams during the day and 500 milligrams at bedtime). A calcium supplement should contain vitamin D (enhances calcium absorption), or be taken with a dairy product. Also, citrus increases calcium absorption, and this supplement can be taken with orange juice.

- If you are eating two servings of calcium from a dairy product, take 500 milligrams of calcium.

Keep a Fat Budget

For most of us, it's just too confusing trying to figure out the percentage of fat calories for a diet. Make your life simple; count fat grams instead. The good news is that chilies will make reducing the amount of fat in your diet easy. Although you will be eating less fat, chilies increase the perception of "oiliness" in carbohydrate foods. Not only will you feel full, you will also feel satisfied—a key component that is often missing in low-fat diets. Within one month, you will crave the clean, spicy and citrus flavors of foods on this program and won't miss the subtle, round flavor of fat. Women should eat no more than 23 grams per day, while men should limit their fat intake to 28 grams of fat per day.

Conquering Trigger Foods

Some people can eat a few potato chips, while others can't stop eating chips until the bag is empty. Before you start the program, go through your cupboards and refrigerator and determine which foods trigger a binge. Chocolate, cheese, cheese pizza, nuts, mayonnaise, salad dressings, fatty red meats, ice cream, cakes and pastries are the most common trigger foods. If you have a history of abusing any of these items, remove them from the house and replace them with healthier alternatives. Until the chilies kick in and you've been on the program for at least one month, the best strategy is to keep these foods out of sight.

TIPS FOR PREVENTING BINGES

- If you nibble while preparing meals, keep a plate of sliced raw vegetables sprinkled with lime juice and chili seasoning next to the stove.
- Plan ahead if you know that you are going to have a stressful week. Keep a supply of healthy, low-fat "binge" food snacks at your office and at home.
- Eat your meals at a dining table. Do not eat in front of the TV or at the vending machine.
- Eat your meals on a salad plate. This will automatically limit the size of your portions.

Trigger Foods	Healthier Alternatives
Potato chips	Baked chips sprinkled with chili seasoning
Tortilla chips	Baked tortilla chips with salsa
Pizza	Armenian pizza bread topped with low-fat cheese, veggies and red pepper
Chocolate	Healthy Choice Fudge Bars, low-fat chocolate pudding
Ice cream	Nonfat frozen yogurt, strawberry gelato
Cheese	Kraft 2% Milk Fat Cheese (slices only)
Mayonnaise	Nonfat breadspreads, Janiecy's low-fat yogurt sauces, low-fat mayo

Blue cheese dressing	Nancy's Healthy Kitchen Lite Blue Cheese Dressing
Butter	I Can't Believe It's Not Butter Spray, Tryson House All Natural Buttery Delite Flavor Spray

CHOOSING A GOAL WEIGHT

The biggest mistake you can make at the start of a diet is setting an unrealistic goal weight. You'll feel defeated before you even begin. Rather than focusing on losing fifty pounds, set a goal of five to ten pounds—even if you want to lose a significantly greater amount of weight. When you divide your weight loss goal into smaller increments, it won't seem so overwhelming. This strategy will not only get you motivated, but keep you motivated. Each time you lose another five pounds, that success will be the driving force that propels you forward to the next goal.

PLATEAUS

Occasionally, your weight loss will slow down or stop. This is called a plateau, and it can last up to several weeks. However, this doesn't mean that the diet is no longer working. Plateaus are a natural part of losing weight—often your body is retaining water. Simply continue to follow the diet and be patient. The pounds will start to fall off again.

I hit a plateau each time I lost twenty pounds and when I was trying to drop the last ten. Several people on the program also experienced a frustrating plateau during the last five or ten pounds. If the weight doesn't budge in three weeks, shake up your routine. Increase the duration of your exercise by upping your exercise time from three times per week to four or five times per week. Increase the intensity of your exercise—swing your arms while walking, or find a route with hills. You can also up your chili intake. This seemed to speed things up. However, you must give your body time to adjust to a new weight. Remember, it took a while to gain the weight, and it will take a while to lose it, too. Just hang in there—it will pass.

SABOTEURS

Often, friends or family members will offer you "treats" while you are trying to lose weight. The best way to deal with this situation is to tell them, "No." But tell yourself, *I choose not to eat this food.*

If a spouse, roommate or significant other continues to eat trigger foods in front of you, enlist his or her support by asking that person to eat these foods away from you for at least one month. It takes twenty-one days to break a habit, and thirty days to establish a new one.

RELAPSES

During the first few months of any weight loss program, it's natural to have a few lapses. The truth is, one scoop of ice cream or a cheeseburger is not going to make you fat. What will hinder your success is if you continue to eat these foods. It's crucial that you learn how to recover from a slip, which prevents a lapse from becoming a relapse.

View a lapse as a learning experience—*not a failure.* Instead of throwing in the towel, ask yourself, *What motivated this slip—hunger or appetite?* If you were hungry, chances are you skipped a meal or forgot to eat chilies. If you were not hungry, you were feeding your emotions instead of your stomach. In that case, look at what triggers you to grab food when you are not truly hungry. Frequently, anger, stress, boredom or being tired is the culprit. I call this "heart hunger," and food will never truly satisfy it. Food is only a temporary salve that masks, but never heals, the pain that you're feeding. When you make that connection, a healthier relationship with food will emerge. Use this experience to gain insight—it's the first step in breaking a self-destructive behavior that does not serve you well.

Lapses can be a useful tool that teaches you the difference between acting and reacting—the dieter's downfall. Post a list of questions on the fridge, and go through this list when you start to feel out of control. This technique forces you to think before you act. Often, that's all it takes to stop a binge in its tracks.

Post this list of questions on the fridge, and go through them when you feel out of control.

- "Am I hungry?'"
- "What am I really feeding—my stomach or my emotions?"
- "Will this food solve my problem?"
- "If eating won't solve my problem, what will?"
- "Do I want this food bad enough to wear it?"
- "Is there a more constructive way to deal with this situation?"
- "What positive steps can I take—eat chilies, take a hot shower, exercise, listen to music or call a friend?"

Ask yourself again, *Do I really want this food?* If you do, then eat it—and savor every bite. Begin by eating a small portion slowly and see if that satisfies you. Instead of wolfing down the whole bag of chips, measure out ten (and throw the rest in the sink). Add chilies to your food—chili seasoning tastes great with a few chips! Go for the regular hamburger, not the Big Mac. Eat three bites of cake, rather than the whole slice. However, if you do eat more than you should, it's important that you do not feel guilty. Just move on, and get back on track with the next meal.

EXERCISE

Unfortunately, we hate to exercise as much as we love to eat. Over 60 percent of Americans don't exercise on a regular basis, while 25 percent don't exercise at all. Moreover, women are more likely to be sedentary than men—by a margin of 49 percent to 33 percent.

Losing weight without exercise is a diet disaster. If you diet without exercise, you'll burn calories from your body's muscle tissue as well as from fat stores. A weight loss of thirty pounds that is half muscle and half fat reduces the muscle mass of the body by fifteen pounds. If you're inactive, that is usually a permanent loss of metabolically active muscle tissue, which translates to a reduced need for calories down the road. Since muscle tissue burns fat at a faster rate than fat tissue (muscle burns fourteen calories per pound over a twenty-four-hour period, while fat tissue only burns two to three calories per pound), the net result of several crash diets can be a lowered metabolism.

The more muscle you have, the easier it will be to lose weight. In addition to burning calories, exercise also helps you lose weight by taming your appetite; it increases levels of the antihunger chemicals dopamine, serotonin, noradrenaline and adrenaline. Moreover, noradrenaline and dopamine double as mood-elevating stimulants. Studies have found that a brisk thirty-minute walk reduces anxiety and can prevent a stress-induced binge. Once you're fit, ten minutes of sustained physical activity can provide an invigorating boost of energy that can last anywhere from six to eighteen hours beyond exercise.

If you hate to exercise, try walking. It's one of the best ways to get fit. It doesn't cost anything, you can do it anywhere, and it's the least likely form of exercise to cause injury. The only equipment you will need is a good pair of walking shoes. Choose a shoe that will stabilize your ankles. Look for a shoe that uses lightweight materials and has a thin heel and flexible toe. (Shoes that have extremely thick soles—aerobic, running shoes and cross-trainers—aren't the best shoes for walking.) Make sure the shoe has a thumb's width from the end of your longest toe to the front of the shoe. If you experience a tingling or numbing sensation in your toes while walking, chances are the toebox in the shoe is too small.

Walking briskly will get you into shape. It will firm up your muscles, help you lose weight—and *keep* it off. Walking also uses your big muscles—those below the waist that make up 75 to 80 percent of your total muscle mass and condition your heart.

Walking exercises the whole body, and the weight you lose is general. How this works is when you use a muscle, or a group of muscles, they send out hormonal signals to your fat cells to release fat, which is then carried by your blood to the working muscles to burn as fuel. In the Chili Pepper Diet, the exercise prescription is simple: Walk at a brisk pace for thirty minutes at the rate of three to four times per week.

If you haven't exercised in a while, the biggest challenge will be to just get moving. Start by walking at a moderate pace for twenty minutes for one week. During the second week, increase your time to thirty minutes. Increase your time gradually—work up to thirty minutes by tacking on an additional five minutes per week. As you get more fit, vary your walks by finding a route that has hills, or add weights. Your exercise regime should first aim to walk thirty minutes per day at the rate of three times per week. After several weeks, up the rate to four days per week.

It's important to warm up and cool down during exercise. This prevents injuries by increasing the temperature in the muscles and enhancing blood flow to the joints and ligaments. The easiest way to warm up is to walk at a slow pace for the first few minutes, then stretch each leg for twenty seconds. Now, pick up the pace—it should be a brisk clip, but not to the point that you are unable carry on a conversation. You should maintain this phase (walking without stopping) for twenty to thirty minutes and break a light sweat.

Cool down by walking slowly for several minutes, then stretch. The key muscles you use during walking are the calves, quadriceps (the muscles in front of your thighs) and hamstrings (the muscles in back of your thighs). Stretch these muscles, followed by your torso, arms and shoulders. Your stretch should be a long and smooth movement that is felt in the muscles (there should be no sensation of pain in your joints). Stretch until you feel tension—not pain—and hold the stretch at that point for about forty-five seconds. Don't bounce. Follow up by stretching the other side of your body.

As you start to feel better, make small changes in your daily routine that automatically ups your activity level. Instead of using the elevator, take the stairs. For instance, if you have an appointment on the sixteenth floor, take the elevator to the fourteenth floor and walk up and down two. If you have a doctor's appointment, make it a habit to park one block away. At the market, find a spot farthest from the entrance, and return the shopping cart to the cart return. And ditch that remote control—get up and change the channel. Over the course of a year, these minor changes add up to a significant number of extra calories (and fat) that your body will burn!

STAYING MOTIVATED

Often, the hardest part of exercise is getting started. Start by laying your exercise clothes out the night before, and put them near the front door. This small act will set the process in motion. When you start to hear the negative thoughts in your head, *I'm just too tired, I don't feel like it, I'll do double time tomorrow,* stop those thoughts in their tracks by repeating to yourself, *This is a gift I give myself.* Use this as your exercise mantra, and keep repeating this phrase as you head out the door. Also, try starting your walk with a prayer. If you set aside this quiet time to talk to God or your higher power, it will give you strength.

The time you select to walk can make a huge difference in how easy it will be to maintain your exercise regime. What's important is to find a time that works for you. Many people find that working out in the morning, or during their lunch break, works for them. Others prefer to work out later in the day. One advantage of working out late in the afternoon, or before dinner, is that it can help you get a more restful sleep. While aerobic exercise initially raises your body temperature and metabolism, by the time you go to bed you experience a drop in body temperature, which makes your sleep deeper and more restorative.

It also helps to schedule your walks with a friend who will hold you to your commitment. However, if you can't find a friend to join you, walk to music—it makes it less boring. Buy a Walkman and keep it with your exercise clothes.

There seems to be a "wall" that exists with exercising—often the first five minutes are the most difficult. However, once you pass that point, you will start to feel energized. Just hang in there—there is a light at the end of the tunnel. Make a mental list of the benefits of exercise: It burns fat; it conditions the heart; it reduces glucose levels; it alleviates stress; it lowers the set point for weight; it makes you more creative; and it keeps you feeling young and strong. Repeat this list to yourself during those first five minutes, and it will carry you through the "wall."

Be fully engaged in the beauty that surrounds you while you're walking. Enjoy the warm feeling of sunlight on your skin, listen to joyful songs of birds and be aware of the intoxicating scents of flowers and freshly mown grass. If you live in a city, pick up on its energy. When you live in the moment, your senses become heightened, you think more clearly and you're left feeling emotionally satisfied.

GETTING BACK ON TRACK

Accept the fact there will be days when you just don't feel like exercising—you're exhausted, you've been out with the flu—whatever. However, don't let a valid reason for not exercising keep you from getting back on track. Start again slowly: Shoot for a ten-minute walk, and work your way back up to a sustained thirty to forty minutes. If you divide your exercise time into smaller segments, it won't seem so overwhelming. Also, give yourself credit for taking a positive step—just getting dressed and heading out the door is a victory when you're not in the mood. Think of fitness as a process, rather than a goal.

Tips for Staying Motivated

- Think of exercise as a gift you give to yourself.
- Start your walk with prayer.
- Exercise with a friend.
- Exercise to music.
- Vary your routine—find routes with hills.
- Be mindful of the beauty of your surroundings as you walk.
- If you just can't do thirty minutes, shoot for three segments of ten minutes.

A Twenty-One Day Meal Plan

Day 1

Breakfast

small bagel with 2 tablespoons
   Caper Cream Cheese Spread (see
   recipe) (or nonfat cream cheese),
   1 oz. smoked salmon and 4 slices
   tomatoes
coffee or tea (no sugar)

1 plum
water
1 ancho chili eaten before the meal
   (or 1 minced jalapeno topping
   bagel)

Mid-morning snack

1 cup strawberries (about 10
   strawberries)

water

Lunch

turkey breast (2 oz.) sandwich on
   whole wheat bread with mustard,
   lettuce, 4 slices tomato, onions and
   1–2 pickled jalapeno peppers
1 cup vegetable soup
   with ¼ tsp. red pepper flakes

1 plum
iced tea (no sugar)
1 cup nonfat milk
water

Dinner

3 oz. roast chicken breast with ⅓ cup
   Cilantro Chutney (see recipe) (or
   salsa of choice)
½ cup Rice Verde (see recipe)

1 cup steamed green beans topped
   with 2 tablespoons of Creamy Light
   Caesar Dressing (see recipe)

Snack

½ cup Strawberry Gelato
   (see recipe)

Day 2

Breakfast

1 cup Oatmeal with Cinnamon and
    Blueberries (see recipe)
1 cup nonfat milk

coffee or tea (no sugar)
water

Mid-morning snack

1 cup strawberries
    (or fruit of choice)

water

Lunch

2 Soft Chicken Tacos (see recipe)
1 cup melon balls
    with fresh lime juice

iced tea (no sugar)
water

Mid-afternoon snack

1 apple
water

1 ancho chili

Dinner

3 oz. roast chicken breast with ⅓ cup
    Cilantro Chutney (see recipe) (or
    salsa of choice)
½ cup Dry Roasted Curried Potatoes
    (see recipe)

1 cup salad plus ½ cup chopped
    vegetables (carrots, onion,
    mushrooms and bell peppers)
    with 2 tablespoons of Creamy Dill
    Dressing (see recipe) (or nonfat
    dressing)
1 ancho chili

Snack

½ mango with fresh lime juice

Day 3

Breakfast

1 cup oatmeal
1 banana
1 cup nonfat milk

coffee or tea (no sugar)
water

Mid-morning snack

1 cup of cantaloupe cubes with fresh
lime juice

water
1 ancho chili

Lunch (restaurant)

3 oz. chicken breast
1 cup pasta with ½ cup marinara
sauce with ¼–½ tsp. red pepper
flakes

1 cup salad with 2 tablespoons nonfat
dressing with 2–4 pickled peppers
iced tea (no sugar)
water

Mid-afternoon snack

1 apple

water

Dinner

Grilled Shrimp with Ancho Chilies
(see recipe)
3 steamed new potatoes (4 oz.)
with ⅓ cup of Cilantro Chutney
(see recipe)

1 steamed artichoke with 2 tablespoons
of Creamy Dill Dressing (see
recipe)

Snack

1 peach

Day 4

Breakfast

Eggs with Mushrooms, Onions and
    Broccoli (see recipe) with
    2 tablespoons El Pato Mexican
    Tomato Sauce (Hot Style) (or ¼ tsp.
    crushed red pepper flakes)

1 slice whole wheat toast
    with 1 tablespoon of Olive Cream
    Cheese Spread (see recipe) and 2
    slices tomato
½ cup nonfat milk
coffee or tea (no sugar)
water

Mid-morning snack

1 pear

water

Lunch

Curried Tuna Salad (see recipe)
3 low-fat whole wheat crackers

iced tea
water

Mid-afternoon snack

1 apple
½ cup nonfat yogurt

water

Dinner

2 Soft Chicken Tacos (see recipe)
Fresh Corn with Lime and
    Chili Seasoning (see recipe)

iced tea
water

Snack

1 plum

Day 5

Breakfast

1 cup Raisin Bran cereal
½ cup nonfat milk
½ pink grapefruit

coffee or tea (no sugar)
water

Mid-morning snack

½ papaya with fresh lime juice
1 ancho chili

water

Lunch

2 Soft Chicken Tacos (see recipe)
2 plums

iced tea (no sugar)
water

Mid-afternoon snack

1 apple
water

1 ancho chili

Dinner

Seared Shrimp with Ancho Chilies
(see recipe)
Fresh Corn with Lime Juice and
Chili Seasoning (see recipe)

1½ cups mixed salad with
2 tablespoons nonfat dressing
of choice

Snack

½ cup low-fat pudding

water

Day 6

Breakfast

2 slices whole wheat toast
   with 2 tablespoons Olive Cream
   Cheese Spread (see recipe) (or
   nonfat cream cheese)
4 slices tomato, 1 pickled pepper

1 egg (poached, soft-boiled or
   hard-boiled)
½ cup nonfat milk
coffee or tea (no sugar)
water

Mid-morning snack

1 banana

water

Lunch

Mexican Chicken Salad with
   Avocado Salsa (see recipe)
1 plum

iced tea
water

Mid-afternoon snack

apple
½ cup nonfat yogurt

1 ancho chili
water

Dinner

Chilean Sea Bass with Tequila Lime
   Sauce (see recipe)
½ cup Rice Verde (see recipe)

1 cup green salad plus ½ cup mixed
   chopped vegetables (carrots, bell
   peppers and tomatoes) with
   2 tablespoons Chili Pepper Diet
   dressing of choice and 2 pickled
   peppers

Snack

½ mango with fresh lime juice

Day 7

Breakfast

1 egg (hard-boiled, soft-boiled or
poached)
1 cup berries
1 slice whole wheat toast
with 1 tablespoon of Olive Cream
Cheese Spread (see recipe)
(or nonfat cream cheese spread)
and 4 slices tomato

coffee or tea
water
1 ancho chili

Mid-morning snack

½ cantaloupe with fresh lime juice

water

Lunch (Subway Restaurant)

1 6-inch turkey sandwich on whole
wheat bread with mustard, 4 slices
tomato, green bell pepper,
1–2 pickled jalapenos, salt,
pepper and oregano (no cheese)

2 plums (or fruit of choice)
diet soda
water

Mid-afternoon snack

1 apple

water

Dinner

Swordfish with Roasted Red Pepper
Sauce (see recipe)

1 cup salad with 2 tablespoons
Creamy Dill Dressing (see recipe)
and 2 pickled peppers
½ cup steamed brown rice with ⅓ cup
Cilantro Chutney (or salsa of
choice) (see recipe)

Snack

½ pink grapefruit

Day 8

Breakfast

1 cup Raisin Bran cereal

½ cup nonfat milk

½ cantaloupe with fresh lime juice

coffee or tea (no sugar)

water

Mid-morning snack

1 pear

1 ancho chili

water

Lunch

bagel with 2 tablespoons nonfat
cream cheese, 2 oz. smoked
salmon, 4 slices tomato, fresh
lemon juice; 1–2 pickled peppers

½ cup fruit salad with fresh lime juice

iced tea

water

Mid-afternoon snack

1 apple

water

Dinner

Chinese Chicken Salad (see recipe)

water

Snack

½ cup Strawberry Gelato (see recipe)

Day 9

Breakfast

1 cup Raisin Bran cereal
1 cup skim milk
1 orange

coffee or tea (no sugar)
water

Mid-morning snack

½ papaya with fresh lime juice

water

Lunch

Vegetarian Burrito (see recipe)
1 plum

iced tea (no sugar)
water

Mid-afternoon snack

1 apple

water

Dinner

Grilled Salmon with Chipotle Cream
(see recipe)
Fresh Corn with Lime and Chili
Seasoning (see recipe)

1 cup steamed green beans
with 2 tablespoons Creamy Dill
Dressing (see recipe) (or low-fat
dressing of choice)

Snack

½ papaya with fresh lime juice

Day 10

Breakfast

2½ to 3-inch whole wheat bagel
    with 2 tablespoons Olive Cream
    Cheese Spread (see recipe) (or
    nonfat cream cheese) and 4 slices
    tomato, 1 pickled jalapeno

1 egg (soft-boiled or hard-boiled)
½ cup nonfat milk
coffee
water

Mid-morning snack

1 orange
water

1 ancho chili

Lunch

½ turkey sandwich with
    4 slices tomato, onion, jalapenos
    and bell peppers on whole wheat
    bread

1 cup vegetable soup
    with ¼ to ½ tsp. red pepper flakes
iced tea
water

Mid-afternoon snack

1 apple
½ cup nonfat yogurt

water

Dinner

3 oz. grilled Atlantic salmon
    with ⅓ cup Cilantro Chutney
    (or salsa of choice) (see recipe)
½ steamed brown rice made
    with sodium reduced chicken stock

1 cup steamed broccoli with
    1 tablespoon of Sesame Ginger
    Salad Dressing (see recipe)
1 ancho chili

Snack

¼ cantaloupe with lime juice

Day 11

Breakfast

Eggs with Mushrooms, Onions and
   Broccoli (see recipe)
1 slice whole wheat toast
   with 1 tablespoon of Olive Cream
   Cheese Spread (see recipe) (or
   nonfat cream cheese) and
   4 slices tomato

½ pink grapefruit
coffee or tea (no sugar)
water

Mid-morning snack

1 pear

1 ancho chili
water

Lunch

Curried Tuna Salad (see recipe)
3 low-fat whole wheat crackers

iced tea
water

Mid-afternoon snack

1 apple

water

Dinner

1½ cups Indian Orange Lentil Soup
   with Ginger and Garlic (see recipe)
1 cup mixed leafy greens, 1–2 pickled
   jalapenos, 1 oz. boiled shrimp and
   2 tablespoons Creamy Dill
   Dressing (see recipe)

1 cup steamed green beans with
   1 ancho chili

Snack

1 cup low-fat yogurt

Day 12

Breakfast

2 slices whole wheat toast
   with 2 tablespoons of Olive Cream
   Cheese Spread (see recipe) (or
   nonfat cream cheese)
4 slices tomato

1 medium egg (soft boiled, poached
   or hard-boiled)
½ pink grapefruit
coffee or tea (no sugar)
1 ancho pepper or 1 pickled jalapeno

Mid-morning snack

½ cantaloupe with fresh lime juice

Lunch

1 cup Progresso Lentil Soup
   with ¼–½ tsp. red pepper flakes
1 cup nonfat yogurt

1 small bag of baby carrots with
   2 tablespoons Creamy Dill Dressing
   (see recipe)
1 plum
iced tea (no sugar)
water

Mid-afternoon snack

1 apple

water

Dinner

Curried Crusted Trout (see recipe)
3 steamed new potatoes (4 oz.)
   with ⅓ cup Cilantro Chutney (see
   recipe) (or salsa of choice)

1 cup steamed green beans
   with 2 tablespoons Creamy
   Dill Dressing (see recipe)
⅔ cup steamed yellow squash

Snack

½ mango with fresh lime juice

Day 13

Breakfast

1 cup oatmeal   coffee or tea
1 cup nonfat milk   water
1 peach

Mid-morning snack

1 banana   water

Lunch

Chinese Chicken Salad (see recipe)   water
iced tea

Mid-afternoon snack

1 apple   water

Dinner

2 Chicken Tacos (see recipe)   1 cup steamed squash with fresh lime
                                         juice and chili seasoning

Snack

½ cup Strawberry Gelato (see recipe)

Day 14

Breakfast

1 cup Raisin Bran
1 cup nonfat milk
½ cantaloupe with fresh lime juice

coffee
water

Mid-morning snack

pear

water
1 ancho chili

Lunch

turkey breast (3 oz.) sandwich on
whole wheat bread with
1 tablespoon Spicy Dijon Spread,
(see recipe) and 1–2 sliced
jalapenos, 4 slices tomato, ½ cup
thinly sliced green bell peppers
and onions

1 cup low-fat tomato soup with
1 teaspoon crushed red pepper
flakes
1 plum
iced tea
water

Mid-afternoon snack

1 apple
1 ancho chili

water

Dinner

Grilled Swordfish with Roasted Red
Pepper Sauce (see recipe)
Fresh Corn with Lime and Chili
Seasoning (see recipe)

1 cup mixed salad greens with
1 jalapeno and 2 tablespoons
nonfat dressing
1 ancho chili

Snack

No evening snack

Day 15

Breakfast

1 egg (hard-boiled, poached or
    soft-boiled)
2 slices whole wheat toast with
    2 tablespoons of Olive Cream
    Cheese Spread (see recipe) (or
    nonfat cream cheese),
    4 slices tomato, 1 jalapeno

1 cup berries
coffee or tea
water

Mid-morning snack

1 orange

1 ancho chili
water

Lunch

1 cup canned fat-free black bean soup
    with ¼–½ tsp. red chili flakes
1 Soft Chicken Taco (see recipe)
1 peach

iced tea
water

Mid-afternoon snack

¾ cup fresh pineapple
    with lime juice

water
1 ancho chili

Dinner

3 oz. Curry Crusted Salmon (see
    recipe)
1 cup steamed broccoli with
    1 tablespoon Sesame Ginger
    Salad Dressing (see recipe)

3 steamed new potatoes (4 oz.)
    with ⅓ cup Cilantro Chutney
    (see recipe)
1 ancho chili

Snack

1 cup nonfat milk

Day 16

Breakfast

1 cup oatmeal

1 cup nonfat milk

¼ cantaloupe with fresh lime juice

coffee or tea

water

Mid-morning snack

1 pear

water

Lunch

1 cup Roasted Poblano Hummus
(see recipe)
with ½ 6-inch pita

½ cup plain, nonfat yogurt

10 baby carrots

1 plum

1 ancho chili

Mid-afternoon snack

1 apple

water

Dinner

4 oz. grilled Atlantic salmon
with ⅓ cup Cilantro Chutney
(see recipe)

Fresh Corn with Lime Juice and
Chili Seasoning (see recipe)

1 cup steamed green beans

water

Snack

½ papaya with fresh lime juice

Day 17

Breakfast

1 cup Raisin Bran cereal

1 cup nonfat milk

½ cup cantaloupe cubes
   with fresh lime juice

coffee or tea

water

Mid-morning snack

10 strawberries

water

Lunch

2 Soft Chicken Tacos (see recipe)

½ cup fruit salad with fresh lime juice

iced tea

water

Mid-afternoon snack

1 cup raspberries

½ cup low-fat yogurt

water

Dinner

3 oz. roast chicken breast with ⅓ cup
   Cilantro Chutney (see recipe)
   (or hot salsa of choice)

½ cup Dry Roasted Curried Potatoes
   (see recipe)

⅔ cup steamed squash with ¼ cup
   low-fat marinara sauce and ¼ tsp.
   red pepper flakes

Snack

½ papaya with fresh lime juice

Day 18

Breakfast

1 cup oatmeal

½ cup nonfat milk

1 orange

coffee or tea

water

Mid-morning snack

1 apple

water

Lunch

2 slices pumpernickel bread
with 2 tablespoons Caper Cream
Cheese Spread (see recipe) (or
nonfat cream cheese),
2 ounces smoked salmon,
4 slices tomato,

5 cucumber slices,
2 minced pickled jalapenos
½ cup fruit salad
iced tea
water

Mid-afternoon snack

1 apple

water

1 ancho chili

Dinner

4 oz. roast turkey breast

3 small boiled new potatoes (4 oz.)
with ⅓ cup Cilantro Chutney
(see recipe)

1 cup steamed mixed vegetables
(broccoli, mushrooms, onions) with
½ teaspoon olive oil
1 cup salad with 2 pickled jalapenos
and 2 tablespoons of low-fat
dressing of choice

Snack

1 plum

Day 19

Breakfast

1 egg (soft-boiled, hard-boiled or poached)

1 2½–3-inch bagel with 2 tablespoons Olive Cream Cheese Spread (see recipe) (or nonfat cream cheese) and 4 slices tomato

¼ cantaloupe with fresh lime juice

1 ancho chili

coffee or tea

water

Mid-morning snack

1 pink grapefruit

water

Lunch

½ turkey breast sandwich on whole wheat bread with 4 slices tomato, sliced green bell peppers, 2 pickled peppers, 2 tablespoons Dijon mustard

1 cup Broccoli Slaw (see recipe)

½ cup plain low-fat yogurt

iced tea

water

Mid-afternoon snack

1 apple

water

Dinner

Goat Cheese Pizza with Olives (see recipe)

1 cup salad plus ½ cup tomatoes, mushrooms, bell peppers, 2 pickled peppers and 2 tablespoons Blue Cheese Dressing (see recipe)

½ cup steamed green beans with fresh lemon juice (ponzu sauce is a light Japanese soy sauce flavored with citrus juice, which can be found at Oriental markets or the condiments section of some supermarkets)

Day 20

Breakfast

1 cup Raisin Bran cereal
1 cup nonfat milk
¼ cantaloupe with fresh lime juice

coffee
water

Mid-morning snack

1 banana

water

Lunch

1 cup Progresso Lentil Soup
   with ½ teaspoon crushed
   red pepper flakes
½ chicken (2 oz. poached or roasted)
   sandwich on whole wheat bread
   with 4 slices tomato, lettuce, sliced
   green bell peppers, onions, 1
   pickled jalapeno and
   1 tablespoon Dijon mustard

¾ cup pineapple with fresh lime juice
iced tea
water

Mid-afternoon snack

1 apple
½ cup low-fat yogurt

water

Dinner

4 oz. grilled Atlantic salmon with ⅓
   cup Red Salsa (see recipe) (or salsa
   of choice)
½ cup Dry Roasted Curried Potatoes
   (see recipe)

1 cup steamed mixed vegetables
   (broccoli, onions and mushrooms)
   with ½ tsp. olive oil)

Snack

No evening snack

Day 21

Breakfast

Oatmeal with Cinnamon and
    Blueberries (see recipe)
½ cup nonfat milk

coffee or tea
water

Mid-morning snack

½ papaya with fresh lime juice

water
1 ancho chili

Lunch

Mexican Chicken Salad with Avocado
    Salsa (see recipe)
1 cup fruit salad with fresh lime juice

iced tea
water

Mid-afternoon snack

½ cup fruit salad
    with fresh lime juice

½ cup nonfat yogurt
water

Dinner

1 Chili Pepper Diet Hamburger
    (see recipe)
½ cup steamed green beans
    with fresh lemon juice
1 cup low-fat tomato soup

with 1 teaspoon red pepper flakes

CHAPTER SEVEN

SMART CHOICES

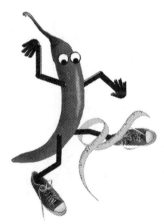

Losing weight begins in those over-lit aisles of your market. If you can't keep that bag of chips out of your cart in the grocery store, what chance do you have of keeping it out of your mouth at home?

Making smart food choices at the market is your first line of defense in the battle of the bulge. Stocking up on great-tasting, low-fat foods will keep you from ordering that pepperoni pizza when you're just too frazzled to cook. Moreover, eating more meals at home gears you toward a healthier diet—you're in control of the quality and quantity of food.

The good news is, if chosen carefully, packaged foods can be part of a healthy diet. Where you run into problems with packaged foods is finding products that are not only healthy—but tasty. While there are some great products that will make losing weight a lot easier, many commercial "diet foods" are Maalox moments. But take heart: The guidelines and products recommended in this chapter will take a lot of the trial and error out of making smart food choices when you're faced with the thirty thousand items a typical supermarket sells.

MARKETING GUIDELINES

Here are some supermarket shopping tips.

- Never shop when you're hungry—you'll be inclined to buy items that are both high in fat and sugar. Make a list, and stick to the list.
- Try to schedule your shopping when stores aren't crowded—the stress of waiting in long checkout lines can be a powerful trigger for buying unnecessary impulse items.
- Pass on products that are high in fat. Generally, products that list oil as one of the first three ingredients should be avoided.
- Limit products that are high in sugar, and use only in small amounts. Sugar can be listed as: sucrose, dextrose, brown sugar, honey, molasses, dextrin, corn syrup, high fructose corn syrup, corn sweeteners, concentrated fruit juice, raw sugar, turbindo sugar, brown rice syrup, barley malt syrup and date sugar.
- Pass on products that list partially hydrogenated oils and/or tropical oils (coconut and palm) on the ingredient list.
- Fresh is best. Take advantage of the seasonal produce, fruits and fish in your area.

HEALTH-FOOD STORES

Not all items sold in health-food stores are worth the extra expense. For instance, granolas are loaded with fat and sweeteners, honey is still sugar, and sea salt is more difficult to use than kosher salt. Not only are these items more expensive, they aren't any healthier.

However, grains and legumes are a better buy in health-food stores than in most supermarkets. These items are sold in bulk so the prices are kept low. Stock up on brown rice, lentils, split peas and beans. You will really notice a difference in the flavor of organic produce, especially apples and potatoes. Buy organic dairy products that don't use hormones or antibiotics. Moreover, health-food stores often carry a better selection of low-fat frozen entrees. I am willing to pay a little more for these items because they are free of partially hydrogenated oils and preservatives.

HOW FOOD LABELS MAKE YOU FAT

Where most of us slip up reading food labels is not checking to see if the serving size listed by the manufacturer is realistic. To keep the fat grams low on the label, food companies divide their products into tiny portions. Don't be fooled by this marketing ploy.

Frequently, you see small serving sizes listed with dips, snack foods and beverages. A prime example is hummus spreads, which list a serving as two tablespoons. Most people would consider the half-cup container a normal portion, downing 400 calories and 24 grams of fat as a snack! You'd be better off eating spicy black bean dip, which is often prepared without added fat. Before you put dips in your cart, ask yourself, "Will I be able to stop at two tablespoons?" If not, don't bring it home.

Watch out for pretzels and crackers as well. Some brands pack up to six grams of fat per handful. Also, many beverages hold two servings, which delivers a double dose of calories and sugar. The label on a sixteen-ounce Snapple lists 110 calories per serving, but the bottle holds two servings, which brings the total calories up to 220. When was the last time you drank half a bottle of Snapple?

LABEL LANGUAGE

Food labels can be a valuable tool for losing weight, but most of us don't know how to read them. And it's not our fault: Some labels are confusing, while others are misleading. That package of ham is labeled "lean," and the mayo is touted as "light." However, one of these "diet foods" packs close to 10 grams of fat per serving.

The "lean" ham can have almost 10 grams of fat in a 3-ounce serving. Although this product is peddled as "lean," almost half (49 percent) of its calories come from fat. Don't rely on marketing terms to make smart food choices. They are merely advertising tags designed to entice you to buy the product.

Although a product may be advertised as "lean" or "extra-lean," that doesn't mean it's low-fat. "Lean" just means it has fewer than 10 grams of fat per serving, while "extra lean" denotes less than 5 grams of total fat in a serving. "Low-fat" translates to no more than 3 grams of total fat per serving.

In the Chili Pepper Diet, the principle item on the food label is the amount of total fat, which is listed in grams. Generally, look for products that have no more than 3 grams of fat per serving. The exceptions are fish, beans, grains and complete frozen entrees, which can have more.

How to Make Smart Food Choices

This three-step process will help you figure out which products can go into your cart, and those that should stay on the shelf.

1. See if the amount of total fat grams is an acceptable number.

2. Check if the listed serving size is realistic.

3. If the listed serving size is small, multiply the total fat grams by the number of servings size you would eat.

Below is a list of commonly used marketing terms that describe packaged products:

- "Fat-Free": contains less than 0.5 grams of total fat per serving.
- "Low-Fat": contains no more than 3 grams of fat per serving.
- "Extra Lean": contains less than 5 grams of total fat, 2 grams of saturated fat and 95 milligrams of cholesterol per 3-ounce serving.
- "Lean": contains fewer than 10 grams of total fat, 4 grams of saturated fat and 95 milligrams of cholesterol per 3-ounce serving.
- "Reduced Fat" or "Less Fat": has 25 percent less fat than the traditional version.
- "Saturated Fat-Free": contains less than 0.5 grams of saturated fat and less than 0.5 grams of trans-fats per serving.
- "Light" or "Lite": contains at least one-third fewer calories or 50 percent less fat than the reference product per 3-ounce serving. However, this vague marketing term may also mean the product is a lighter color or has less weight. Read the label.
- "Calorie-Free": contains less than 5 calories per serving.

- "Low-calorie": contains less than 40 calories per serving.
- "No sugar added": means there's no table sugar added. However, it may contain other forms of sugar—corn syrup, fructose, glucose and sucrose.
- "Natural": means the product has no additives or artificial ingredients. However, a "natural" product can be full of fat and sugar.
- "Natural" (meat): the product is free of additives, such as sugar, preservatives and colorings. This term does not designate that the meat was organically grown (without drugs or antibiotics).

WHAT FOOD LABELS DON'T TELL YOU

There is no legal mandate that requires companies to list trans-fats on the label. However, if a product has "partially hydrogenated oils" on the ingredient list, it indicates that trans-fats are present. To avoid this artery-clogging fat, pass on products that have "hydrogenated oils" or "partially hydrogenated oils." Even if the Nutrition Facts lists 0 grams of fat, that does not mean the product is trans-fat free—it means it has less than 0.5 grams per serving. By the time you polish off the entire container, you will have eaten a lot of the wrong kind of fat.

Remember, the harmful effects of trans-fats are just as bad, if not greater, than those produced by saturated fats. Saturated fats increase both total cholesterol and LDL cholesterol (the bad kind). However, trans-fats not only increase total cholesterol and LDL cholesterol but decrease HDL cholesterol (the good kind). Trans-fats unfavorably affect the enzymes used for fat metabolism, and alter the number and size of fat cells. Finally, trans-fats deplete omega-3 fatty acids (the good-for-your-heart oils), and decrease the insulin response, which is undesirable for diabetics.

Don't switch from saturated fats to products that contain partially hydrogenated oils to lose weight—it's a bad trade-off. Ten years of nondairy creamer in your coffee, light microwave popcorn for snacks, broccoli in low-fat cheese sauce on your baked potatoes and frozen dinners could very well be at the expense of your heart. An epidemiologist at Harvard Medical School, Mathew Gillman, analyzed the data on 832 men whose diets had been tracked for over twenty-one years, and what he uncovered was shocking—men who ate 5 teaspoons or more of margarine per day had nearly twice the rate of heart problems than those who abstained. Clearly, the harmful effects of trans-fats are unmatched to any kind of natural fatty acid.

Trans-fats appear in almost every kind of processed food: light microwave popcorn, nondairy creamers, crackers, cereals, frozen entrees, margarine, breads, sauces, sauce mixes, pancake mixes, vanilla and chocolate milk mixes, sport/supplement bars, diet bars, fruit snacks, flavored instant coffee mixes, cereal bars, "low-fat" cookies, pastries, "fat-free" candies, pie crusts, cake mixes, "low-fat" puddings and nondairy whipped toppings.

Researchers estimate the average American eats anywhere from 5.3 grams up to 12 grams of trans-fat per day. Processed foods using partially hydrogenated oils contribute 80 percent of that amount. According to researcher Dr. Udo Erasmus, "Margarine accounts for 3.5 grams, while shortenings contribute 4.6 grams. Salad oils add 0.5 grams per day."

However, trans-fats also occur naturally in meat and dairy products. Currently, researchers estimate that about a fifth of the trans-fats in our diets come from animal products. So, when you choose to eat dairy or beef, make it count.

Frozen Foods

Without a doubt, fresh vegetables have the best flavor. However, many of us just don't have the time or talent to cook them properly. If you're one of the culinarily challenged, stock up on frozen vegetables, which tend to have fewer additives and less sodium than complete dinners. These products are great time-savers since the labor-intensive prep work has been done. And next to doing the dishes, no other job keeps more people out of a kitchen than washing, peeling and chopping veggies. Moreover, frozen vegetables are a smarter choice than canned because they retain more nutrients.

The freezing process will rob vegetables of their crunch, so be careful that you don't overcook them. Using quick-cooking methods, such as lightly stir-frying and blanching, will make the difference between these products being a reasonably good side dish and that "mess that goes to the dog." Also, some vegetables seem to weather the freezing process better than others—peas, flash-frozen green beans and stir-fry medleys seem to do the best.

Frozen Entrees

Unfortunately, partially hydrogenated oils show up in many of the frozen entrees peddled to the weight-loss market. Another problem with complete dinners is they taste bland. At best, the majority of frozen entrees I've tried taste like airline food. I don't know how they do it, but food companies manage to process out all of the flavor and texture in any food they touch. Most of the time, I can't tell where the overcooked rice ends and the mushy chicken begins. As for pasta dinners, have these companies ever heard of "al dente"?

Ethnic Gourmet sells a variety of excellent frozen entrees that have a moderate fat level, contain no additives, are well-spiced and use fiber-rich brown rice. And best of all, they taste great! Stouffer's and Weight Watchers are worth a try, but be sure to read the labels—some entrees contain partially hydrogenated oils, while others are low in protein and fiber.

However, if you're hungry, even a tasty 300-calorie complete dinner will not fill you up. The major drawback to this type of product is small serving sizes. Fortunately, you can easily solve this problem by teaming them up with a small salad (seasoned with fresh lemon juice and chilies) and a glass of nonfat milk. As a general rule, try to limit yourself to two entrees per week, and make up the bulk of your diet from freshly prepared foods.

Since new products are hitting the market all the time, I've listed a few guidelines for making smart choices when grabbing frozen entrees:

- No hydrogenated oils.
- Limit total fat to 7 grams per serving.
- Has no less than 3 grams of fiber.
- Has at least 10 grams of protein per serving (shoot for 13 to 19 grams).
- Product has minimal additives.

TIP: For some unknown reason, poultry, pasta and bean-based dishes seem to weather the freezing process better than fish and beef.

Product	Calories	Fat	Fiber	Protein
Taj Gourmet Chicken Tandoori w/Vegetables	320	6 g	5 g	19 g
Palak Paneer (Spinach w/homemade cheese)	320	7 g	7 g	13 g
Chicken Tandoori w/Spinach	330	7 g	5 g	20 g
Chicken Tikka Masala Wrap	320	7 g	3 g	17 g
Stouffer's Lean Cuisine Three Bean Chili	250	6 g	10 g	10 g

VEGGIE BURGERS

Although food companies market veggie patties as an alternative to "burgers," these products do not taste like meat. Nor will they satisfy a craving for beef. However, that does not mean they don't taste good. And chances are, if you like the taste of falafel balls, you'll keep this product stocked in your freezer. In fact, veggie burgers are one of the tastiest ways to introduce the Western palate to soy.

There are many brands of veggie burgers to choose from, and frankly, some taste better than others. Also, patties deliver a wide range in grams of protein; choose a brand that has at least 10 grams.

Product	Calories	Fat	Fiber	Protein	Taste
Boca Burger	90	0.5 g	4 g	11 g	Has a "meaty" texture
Morning Star Farms Garden Veggie Patties	100	2.5 g	4 g	10 g	Tastes "fried," crunchy veg-etables add a nice flavor and texture

PASTA SAUCES

You can't go wrong nutritionally with these tomato-based sauces: They are low in fat, are a good source of vitamin A and are packed with lycopene, the phytochemical that appears to protect against prostate cancer.

Supermarket aisles are jammed with gourmet pasta sauces. Most markets carry at least eight different brands. Which one do you choose, and how do they taste? Buy several brands and rotate between them.

Classico's Tomato & Basil is a good sauce that delivers 1 gram of fat per serving. However, its flavor is a tad bland. Use this sauce as a base, and add fresh herbs, mushrooms and tomatoes. Barilla makes a wonderful pasta sauce, Green & Black Olive, that delivers a great "olive" taste at only 2.5 grams of fat per serving. You don't need to add anything to this sauce—just pour it out of the jar. The only draw-back to this product is it is high in sodium, so pass on this product if you're sodium sensitive. The best tomato sauce on the market is Roa's

Homemade Marinara sauce—hands down. It has the best vine-ripened tomato flavor. However, this sauce contains more olive oil, so reserve it for special occasions.

Product	Serving Size	Calories	Total Fat	Sodium
Classico Tomato & Basil	½ cup	50	1 g	390 mg
Barilla Green & Black Olive	½ cup	80	2.5 g	1,010 mg
Roa's Homemade Marinara	½ cup	60	4 g	375 mg

DAIRY PRODUCTS

Dairy products are rich in calcium, and that's not just good for your bones—it might also help you lose weight! Recent studies have shown that diets high in calcium keep you thin by changing the way your body processes fat. Just make sure it's low in fat.

Substitute nonfat milk products for whole milk products. If you don't like the "watery" taste of nonfat milk, add one tablespoon of nonfat dry milk powder to your glass of skim milk. It changes the color from "blue" to "white," gives it a richer taste and ups the calcium content. It will take about three weeks for your taste buds to adjust from whole milk to skim milk—just hang in there.

Switch from half & half to Land O' Lakes Fat-Free Half & Half. It really does taste like the real thing. Another alternative to cream (and non-dairy creamers) is evaporated skim milk. Its slightly sweet and rich texture makes it ideally suited for coffee and tea.

Try 1 percent buttermilk in your homemade salad dressings where a tart taste is an advantage. Reserve 1 percent fat milk for recipes that need a touch of richness. A quarter cup of 1 percent milk can really make the difference in both the texture and taste of a low-fat "cream" soup.

SOUR CREAM

In recipes calling for regular sour cream, substitute nonfat sour cream or plain nonfat yogurt. To thicken a sauce or soup made with these products, add a slurry of water and cornstarch at the end of the cooking process. (If you use it during the cooking process, it thins out.) A good ratio is a half-cup of water to one tablespoon of cornstarch. It's a good idea to keep a prepared cornstarch slurry in your refrigerator.

Occasionally, use small amounts of light sour cream or crema Mexicana (table cream) to add richness, or offset the sour taste of nonfat yogurt–based sauces. Light sour cream works better in recipes that contain large amounts of liquid, such as soups and cream-based pasta dishes. Crema Mexicana has a richer, smoother texture that is more suited to sauces. However, be sure to limit the portion size to one tablespoon. Don't confuse Mexican table cream with a similar product, Mexican sour cream (agria), which is high in fat. Always read the label.

Product	Serving	Calories	Fat	Sat. Fat
Crema Mexicana (agria)	2 tbs.	80	8 g	5 g
Knudson Regular Sour Cream	2 tbs.	60	6 g	3.5 g
Low-Fat Alternatives				
Knudson Light Sour Cream	2 tbs.	40	2.5 g	1.5 g
Crema Mexicana (table cream)	1 tbs.	30	2.5 g	1.5 g
Knudson Nonfat Sour Cream	2 tbs.	30	0 g	0 g

CHEESE

Like chocolate, cheese is one of those foods we love and crave. Cheese shows up in salads, sandwiches, burgers, pizza and every snack food you can imagine. In 1999, the average American ate thirty pounds of cheese—that translates to over two pounds per month. Unfortunately, cheese gives us more artery-clogging saturated fat than any other food—even beef. If cheese is a food you can't live without, switch to a fat-reduced cheese for texture and use strong cheeses for flavor.

Nonfat Cheese

If you want to kick your cheese habit, I can't think of a better way to do it than eating a nonfat cheese: They taste like plastic, don't melt and develop a rubbery texture when they cool down. According to cheese manufacturers, it seems the threshold for reducing the fat is about 50 percent. Anything lower than that, and cheese loses the sensual qualities that make it the sinful indulgence we crave.

When too much fat is removed from cheese, the proteins come to the foreground, which can taste bitter and don't melt. Proteins are also responsible for the rubbery texture of nonfat cheese. While making a full-fat cheese is a very complex process, creating a good nonfat cheese is an art—it requires a certain pH and just the right mixture of skim milk proteins to create a product that melts.

One of the best nonfat cheeses on the market is put out by Lifetime, and their cheddar, mozzarella and hickory-smoked mozzarella do work in certain dishes, such as scrambled eggs. However, I don't recommend that you eat them alone—even the best nonfat cheese is a disappointment on a cracker. The *only* way to use a nonfat cheese is to mix it with other ingredients, which masks their texture and flavor.

Cooking with nonfat cheese requires more effort, but it's worth it. First and foremost, nonfat cheeses perform best in dishes with moisture and a little fat. In fact, the secret to using nonfat cheese is *moist* heat, which helps it melt. To create moisture, add a few tablespoons of water near the end of the cooking process and cover the pan to retain the steam. Also, nonfat cheeses melt best if they're chilled, rather than room temperature.

Another trick that creates moisture (and flavor) is placing toppings over the nonfat cheese. One of the best toppings to use with nonfat cheese is minced chives. They not only help it melt but improve its taste. Another topping that works is minced pickled peppers. Also, several sprays of Roasted Garlic Juice by Garlic Valley Farms do wonders to enhance the taste of nonfat cheese. You can find this product in the produce section of your market.

Depending on the recipe, you'll need to use different heat levels to create a quick and even melt. In omelets, use a medium-low heat since nonfat cheese takes longer to melt. In a sauce, add the cheese to boiling liquids. If you follow the guidelines listed below, chances are you'll end up with a dish that's not only healthy, but tasty. (Depending on the manufacturing process, nonfat cheese can have almost twice the amount of calcium as a full-fat cheese.)

Nonfat Cheese Guidelines

- Use a good quality nonfat cheese. Try Lifetime's cheddar, mozzarella and smoked mozzarella.
- Steer clear of the sharp cheddar, jalapeno and Swiss nonfat cheeses—they have an aftertaste.
- Reserve nonfat cheeses for dishes with moisture.
- Use nonfat cheese chilled or frozen—you'll get a better melt.
- Place toppings over nonfat cheese.
- Season nonfat cheese. For example, use several sprays of roasted garlic juice and moist toppings (minced pickled jalapeno peppers and/or minced green onions).
- In egg dishes, add one to two tablespoons of water near the end of the cooking process, and cover pan to conserve steam (steam facilitates the melting process). Use a medium-low heat because nonfat cheese takes longer to melt.
- In cheese sauces, add nonfat cheese to boiling 1 percent low-fat milk to get a quick and even melt.

TIP: Store individual (1 oz.) portions of grated nonfat cheese in your refrigerator or freezer.

LOW-FAT CHEESE AND STRONG-FLAVORED CHEESE

Although it's a healthier choice to eat nonfat cheese, it's not always a smarter choice—most people who rely on these products don't stick with them. While a nonfat Jack will pass (barely) in a spicy bean burrito, it's still a compromise you might not be willing to make. In that case, either eliminate cheese from your recipe, or use small amounts of a fat-reduced or strong flavored cheese instead.

Although parmesan and romano aren't less fatty than other cheeses, they do have more flavor so you can use smaller portions without feeling deprived. One (grated) tablespoon is all it takes to give that plate of pasta a burst of flavor. That amount translates to just 1.5 grams of fat. It works!

Another cheese that works well in small portions is cotija. Although it's made from cow's milk, this marvelous Mexican cheese has a sharp flavor and texture that's reminiscent of a Greek (dry) feta. Cotija cheese is sold in three forms: blocks, wheels and powdered. Look for the crumbled (powdered) version; you can easily portion control it to one tablespoon right from the package.

However, if you're craving the velvety texture of warm, melting cheese, eating grated Parmesan won't cut it. Switch to a fat-reduced cheese instead. Fortunately, refined processing techniques have greatly improved the quality of these products. Sargento Light Deli Style Mozzarella Reduced Fat Cheese slices and Kraft 2% Milk Fat Cheese come pretty close to traditional products in taste and texture. And, yes—they *do* melt.

MAKING CHEESE WORK IN A LOW-FAT DIET

Figure out which sensual quality of cheese you're craving, and then satisfy *that* craving. If you're craving the *texture* of warm melting cheese, use a fat-reduced cheese. If your meal needs a burst of *flavor*, go for the strong-flavored cheeses instead. Remember, you're less likely to go for seconds (and thirds) if you feel satisfied. The caveat with cheese on the Chili Pepper Diet is to use cheeses that contain fat on an occasional basis, and limit your total fat grams to 2.5 grams per serving. Enjoy every bite—make it count!

Cheeses That Work in a Low-Fat Diet

Depending on the recipe, you may need to reduce your serving size to half a slice or half an ounce to keep the fat grams low.

Product	Serving Size	Total Fat
Melting Cheeses		
Sargento, Low-Fat Mozzarella	½ oz.	1.5 g
Kraft 2% Milk Fat Cheese	½ slice	1.5 g
Nonfat Cheese		
Lifetime, Cheddar & Mozzarella	1 oz.	0 g
Spreadable Cheeses		
Philadelphia, Light, tub	1 tbs.	2.5 g
Noah's Light Cream Cheeses	1 tbs.	2.5 g
Nonfat Cream Cheese	2 tbs	0 g
Friendship Spreadable (1% Milkfat) Whipped Low-Fat Cottage Cheese	½ cup	1 g
Strong-Flavored Cheeses		
Parmesan, regular, grated	1 tbs.	1.5 g
Cotija, regular, powdered	1 tbs.	2 g
Feta cheese, regular, crumbled	1 tbs.	1.0 g

BREADS

Most white breads contain less than one gram of fiber per serv-ing—and that's not enough. Switch to a high-fiber bread. Not only do these breads have more flavor, they keep you from feeling hungry for longer periods of time. Whether you choose wheat, oat, pumper-nickel or rye, check the label to see if the word "whole" is the first word in the ingredient list. This ensures you're getting a high-fiber product.

Also, stock up on bagels, corn tortillas and pita breads. These products contain one gram of fiber per serving—double the amount found in white bread. Listed below are several types of breads that are smarter food choices than conventional white bread. If you're hooked on muffins, try Nature's Path Carrot and Raisin Manna Bread. This wonderful Canadian import has a sinfully rich, moist tex-ture that comes close to a dessert. While many bran muffins contain at least seven grams of fat, this product contains no fat.

Product	Fat	Fiber
White Bread	0 g	.5 g
Whole Wheat Bread	1–2.5 g	1–3 g
Pita Bread	0 g	1 g
Corn Tortilla	1 g	1 g
Bagels	1 g	1 g
Nature's Path Manna Bread	0 g	5 g
Mestemacher German Whole Rye	1 g	6 g

PIZZA

A slice of cheese pizza at your local pizzeria runs 14 grams of fat. Celeste's frozen cheese pie for one packs 19 grams of fat. These are hardly the numbers you'd like to see when you're trying to lose weight. If you thought you had to give up pizza because it makes you fat, your ship has just come in.

Trader Joe's Market and Sevan Bakery put out wonderful products, Low-Fat Thin Crust Pizzas, that deliver the taste of fresh pizza at only 2 grams of fat. The only thing that's missing is the toppings and cheese. Top the Hot Tomato & Onion Thin Crust Pizza with a small amount of low-fat mozzarella, sliced veggies and crushed red pepper flakes, and your fresh pizza comes in at 5.5 grams of fat. You can find this product in the bread section at Whole Foods Market, in the refrigerated section at Trader Joe's Market, Costco or in Armenian markets.

SALAD DRESSINGS

Most commercial low-fat salad dressings are Maalox moments— either they taste too sweet or have a harsh vinegary flavor. However, the products listed below prove you really can take out the fat without sacrificing taste.

Calabasas Gourmet Wild Berry and Sage Grilling Sauce and Salad Dressing

This sublime sauce can raise a humble meal to a state of grace. Its brilliant pairing of red wine, berries and sage creates a complexity of flavors rarely seen in a commercial dressing. It works equally well as a marinade, or drizzled over fruit salads or tossed greens. Reduce it with black pepper and juniper berries to create a savory sauce for poultry. And you're not going to believe these numbers—it has a mere seventeen calories and zero grams of fat per tablespoon!

Nancy's Healthy Kitchen Sesame Ginger Dressing

This exotic Asian-inspired dressing combines ginger, pineapple, sesame seeds, garlic and chilies to create a sweet and tangy flavor. And it does all that with only one gram of fat per tablespoon! This product is sweet, so use it on an occasional basis.

Nancy's Healthy Kitchen Lite Blue Cheese Dressing

This product delivers all the tangy flavor of a blue cheese dressing, but at a fraction of the fat with less than two grams of fat per serving. To thicken its texture, add several tablespoons of Friendship Spreadable (1% Milkfat) Whipped Low-Fat Cottage Cheese.

CANNED BEANS

Unlike canned vegetables, canned beans retain most of their nutrients and texture. Another advantage to canned beans is that they don't produce the amount of intestinal gas that cooked dried beans do—the canning process removes most of the gas-causing sugars. The only drawback to canned beans is that they are high in sodium. If you need to watch your sodium intake, drain the beans in a colander and rinse them with cold water. Rinsing canned beans will reduce the sodium content by one-third. If you are not sodium-sensitive, incorporate the liquid into your recipe—it contains fiber. My favorite brand of canned beans is Sun Vista; they have a creamy texture without being mushy.

CHICKEN BROTH

One of the best ways to slash the fat in your diet without sacrific-ing taste is substituting chicken broth for oil when your sautéing food. My favorite canned brand is Swanson 99% Fat-Free Chicken Broth—it has the best chicken flavor. Buy the large cans for soups. For sauces, the most convenient version is packaged in a carton with flip-top opening, which allows you to use small amounts and put the remainder in the refrigerator. Imagine Natural Organic Free Range Chicken Broth has a richer, "homemade" chicken flavor and almost half the sodium of most canned products. I think it's the best product on the market.

FRUIT SPREADS

Substitute all-fruit jams for fatty margarine and butter on your toast or bagel. The best product on the market is the French import St. Dalfour, which uses a slow-cooking reduction technique to con-centrate flavor. This product line is free of artificial colorings and preservatives. And, best of all—it really does taste like Grandma's homemade preserves.

FISH

Select fatty, coldwater fishes, which contain larger amounts of heart-healthy omega-3 oils. Some of the fishes you should try are: salmon, tuna, mackerel, Chilean sea bass and herring. If you're new to fish, start with Atlantic or Norwegian salmon. It has a rich, mild flavor, and a velvety texture that most people just love. Choose a center cut, which has a higher fat content than tail pieces. Atlantic salmon is available year-round in most supermarkets.

Another advantage of salmon is that it's hard to ruin it. It tolerates "overcooking" better than other types of fish. Believe it or not, a great way to cook fish is in a microwave oven—it seals in the moisture so the fish doesn't end up tough and dry. If you're broiling it, cook the salmon skin side up to keep the flesh moist. Remove the skin before eating.

The easiest way to reduce the size of your portions is to stop buying large pieces. Instead, have the fish monger cut four-ounce portions, and wrap them up individually to store in your freezer. Even in markets where the fish is packaged in large pieces, just ring the bell and ask for the fish to be weighed and cut into smaller portions. This automatically portion controls your fish to just the right amount. (Since fish has a high water content, it can lose up to one and a half ounces during cooking.)

If fresh fish is unavailable in your area, stock up on canned salmon and tuna. Be sure the fish is packed in water, not oil. Another alternative to fresh fish is smoked fish. However, pass on any product that lists nitrates on the ingredient list—this preservative has been linked to cancer. A smarter choice is to select a product that uses natural wood smoke as a preservative. Not only is this a healthier product, it has a better flavor and texture. If you have a Costco in your area, Kirkland Signature Label sells a good imported smoked Norwegian salmon at a very reasonable price.

When buying fish, make sure it looks fresh. The flesh should be shiny and firm. When pressed, the flesh should spring back immediately. Check for any yellow or brown discolorations, and make sure there is no darkening on the edges of the fish. Also, fresh fish has a mild smell—never "fishy." Pass on any fish that smells like ammonia. (Unfortunately, you might not detect an ammonia smell until you cook it.)

Shellfish is a good source of protein and low-fat. A recent study uncovered that shrimp may increase levels of HDL cholesterol (the good kind). Choose Mexican whites or Gulf whites that are labeled "15-30"—they have sweetest flavor. Lobster and crab taste best when are purchased live.

Mollusks, such as clams, mussels and oysters, should be purchased live. All mollusks spoil rapidly, and should be used immediately after purchase.

Go Fish

Fish (3-ounce serving)	Omega-3s (g)	Fat (g)
Atlantic salmon	1.5 g	7.0 g
Pink salmon (canned)	1.5 g	5.1 g
Bluefin tuna	1.0 g	4.2 g

IMITATION CRAB

Although imitation crab (surimi) looks like a smart choice on the label (low in fat and high in protein), pass on this product. It has been stripped of all the healthy fish oils. To manufacture this product, the fish (usually pollack) must be bleached before it's formed into a tasteless paste. As it's shaped into strips, artificial colors, sugar and flavors are added to make it palatable. Do not substitute this product for shellfish or fish.

MARGARINE

Next to shortening, the largest contributor of trans-fats in our diets is margarine. Stick margarines have the greatest amount of trans-fats, about 24 percent. Tub margarines contain about 15 percent. Products that are packaged in squeezeable containers (are liquid) contain the least amount of trans-fats.

None of these products were used in the Chili Pepper Diet. Light margarines tend to have a "chemical" taste that most people won't tolerate. You're better off using flavorful low-fat bean spreads or all fruit jams on your toast instead. Moreover, most of these products are not recommended for cooking or baking. Use nonstick butter-flavored sprays for cooking—you'll get better results and use less fat.

POULTRY

Without the skin to protect it, poultry meat dries out when it's cooked. The secret for keeping skinless meat moist is to spray it with a nonstick spray before you bake, broil, sauté or stir-fry. Another technique is to gently poach poultry meat in stock or water, then add it at the end of a recipe.

Skinless chicken breast tenders are ideal for Asian stir-fry dishes. However, this cut of meat will dry out on a hot barbecue. It's better to grill the meat with the skin on (bone side down), then remove the skin before you eat it. Although this technique will add 1 gram of fat, it's worth it. Just subtract that fat from somewhere else in the meal.

Be sure to read the label when you buy ground turkey; many products pack up to 8 grams of fat in a 3-ounce serving. This amount of fat indicates that thigh meat has been mixed in with breast meat. To ensure that you're getting a truly lean product, pick out a breast, and ask the butcher to remove the skin before he runs it through the meat grinder. For added convenience, ask the butcher to wrap it up in individual 3.5-ounce portions.

The secret for cooking juicy, lean turkey burgers: Spray the meat (not the pan) with a nonstick flavor mist, then quickly cook the meat at a high heat to seal in the juices. The nonstick pan must be hot before you add meat—preheating for about a minute should do it. However, do *not* leave a nonstick pan over a hot flame for over five minutes—the coating will release fumes that can irritate your eyes, nose and throat. It's also crucial that you don't overcook the meat, or it will dry out and be tough. The best product for this cooking technique is Tryson House All Natural Mesquite Mist Flavor Spray.

By removing the skin, you'll significantly reduce the amount of fat. Spray skinless poultry with a nonstick flavor spray before cooking to keep it moist.	Calories	Total Fat	Sat. Fat
Chicken (fryer, 3.5 ounces, uncooked)			
Breast, without skin	110	1.2 g	0.3 g
Drumstick, without skin	119	3.4 g	0.8 g
Thigh, without skin	119	3.9 g	1.0 g
Breast, with skin	172	9.2 g	2.6 g
Dark meat, with skin	253	15.8 g	4.4 g
Turkey (young tom, 3.5 ounces, uncooked)			
Light meat, without skin	114	1.5 g	0.5 g
Light meat, with skin	156	6.9 g	.5 g
Dark meat, without skin	124	4.3 g	1.4 g
Dark meat, with skin	159	8.7 g	2.6 g

MEAT

Red meat can be part of a low-fat diet. If you select the leanest cuts of meat and trim away all visible fat (including white connective tissue), meat is lighter than a skinless chicken drumstick. However, meat should be an occasional treat, and limit your portion sizes to 3.5 ounces uncooked.

Choose "select," "round," "rump" and "sirloin tip" cuts of beef for less fat, and use super-lean (5 percent fat) ground beef for burgers. While many cookbooks advocate slow-cooking techniques for lean meat, I've had better results searing it at a high heat, which seals in the juices. To make the most out of small portions of meat, combine it with vegetables and grains. Asian stir-fry dishes are ideal.

Ask your butcher to trim all visible fat and wrap up individual 3.5-ounce portions. The exception to this rule is super-lean ground beef (5 percent fat), in which you can use use 4-ounce portions for burgers. To tenderize lean cuts of meat, marinate them in Asian marinades, fruit juices, flavored vinegars, seasoned nonfat yogurt or red wine and chili for at least two hours (don't exceed twenty-four hours).

The Leanest Meats

	Calories	Total Fat	Sat. Fat
Beef (select grade, trimmed, 3.5 ounces, uncooked)			
Top round	120	2.5 g	0.8 g
Tip round	119	3.2 g	1.0 g
Eye of round	124	3.6 g	1.3 g
Sirloin	124	3.7 g	1.3 g
Super-lean ground beef (5% fat), 4 ounces, uncooked	141	4.5 g	1.5 g
Lamb (choice grade, trimmed, 3.5 ounces, uncooked)			
Leg	128	4.5 g	1.6 g
Pork (trimmed, 3.5 ounces, uncooked)			
Tenderloin	120	3.4 g	1.1 g

MAYONNAISE

One tablespoon of regular mayonnaise packs 11 grams of fat. Switching to light mayonnaise will reduce that number to 5 grams of fat. However, there are better products that deliver a rich, creamy "homemade" taste at only 2.5 grams of fat—per 2 tablespoons!

Janiecy's Tzatziki Creamy Cucumber Garlic Sauce and Creamy Curry Sauce are superb products. They use plain low-fat yogurt as a base, and add a small amount of sour cream to offset the tart taste. The Creamy Curry Sauce has a rich, curry flavor that ends with a nice kick. Pair it with seafood or veggie burgers, and you'll feel totally indulged.

The Tzatziki Sauce uses fresh garlic, dill, onion, lemon juice and cucumber to create a refreshing taste that wakes up any sandwich. The only caveat with these products is to use them chilled—if you heat them, they break down and lose their rich, creamy texture.

Nonfat Mayonnaise

While this product is inedible on its own, you can mix it with other ingredients to create a good tasting product. Use the nonfat mayo as a base, and add strong flavored ingredients (pickled chilies, chili sauces and Dijon mustard), which improves the flavor and texture.

Product	Serving Size	Calories	Total Fat	Sat. Fat
Mayonnaise, regular	1 tbs.	100	11 g	1.5 g
Low-Fat Alternatives				
Mayonnaise, Best Foods, nonfat	1 tbs.	12	0 g	0 g
Janiecy's, Tzatziki Sauce	2 tbs.	35	2.5 g	1.5 g
Janiecy's, Creamy Curry Sauce	2 tbs.	35	2.5 g	2 g
Dijon mustard	1 tbs.	15	0 g	0 g

SALSAS

Many markets carry freshly prepared salsas. Choose products that don't use preservatives; they have a more "homemade" flavor and a better texture. You can "freshen" them up with a squeeze of fresh lemon or lime juice before serving.

You should also have a few canned salsa products on hand. Some of the best products come from Mexico. El Pato's Salsa de Chile Fresco (Tomato Sauce Mexican Hot Style) combines tomatoes, onions, chilies, garlic and spices—no preservatives. You can use it straight from the can as a cooking sauce, or add fresh cilantro for a quick salsa. Pepper's Unlimited Inc. puts out a wonderful Chipotle Sauce that's ready to use right from the can.

Another good Mexican import is Herdez's Salsa Verde, which uses tomatillos, onions, serrano peppers, salt and cilantro. Add fresh minced serrano chilies and cilantro, and this sauce could pass for "homemade." Both products can be found in Latin markets, or ordered online at *www.monterreyfoodproducts.com*. If you live in an area with a large Latin population, check the ethnic section of your supermarket.

La Victoria's Red Salsa Jalapena (extra hot) has a good flavor and a nice kick. If you want sauce with less heat, try Pace's Salsa Picante. Puree these sauces in a blender to improve their texture.

HOT SAUCES

Sriracha Chinese hot sauce has the perfect blend of hot and sweet flavors that complements Chinese and Korean food. Look for it in the ethnic section of your market (it's packaged in a squeezeable plastic bottle). Be sure to pick up one of our own native Louisiana hot sauces—Crystal and Tabasco are excellent products.

MARINADES

A good marinade doesn't need to rely on oil or sugar for flavor—choose a product that is based on fruit juices and chilies instead. Uncle Bum's Hot Jamaican Marinade* combines peppers, lime juice, onion, garlic and spices to create a complex and spicy flavor that works equally well with chicken, meat or fish. Add fresh lime juice and Meyer's dark rum to freshen up its taste. (The alcohol adds flavor and will burn off during cooking.)

Fontera's Smoky Chipotle and Garlic Grilling Sauce works wonders on shrimp and chicken. This rich tomato-based sauce uses lots of fresh garlic, smoky chipotle chilies and just a touch of brown sugar.

CHILI SEASONINGS

Chef Merito's sells two excellent seasoning mixes: Salt, Lemon and Chili and Pikos Picosos. The Salt, Lemon and Chili mix contains salt, powdered lemon juice and chilies, and works best on melons, cucumbers and jicama. Pikos Picosos uses ground chilies and salt (no lemon), and has a lot more heat. Use Pikos Picosos in a pico de gallo–type salad. You can find these products in a Latin market.

Also try Chef Paul Prudhomme's Seafood Magic Seasoning Blend—it's great on fish, steamed vegetables and poultry.

SALAD-IN-A-BAG

Washed, trimmed and bagged fresh salad mixtures and vegetables are great time-savers. When choosing a salad mixture, let color be your guide. Look for mixtures that are based on dark-colored greens, such as romaine or a mixture of dark-colored lettuces. Pass on products that contain preservatives. Add minced carrots with

*This product is sold primarily to hotels and restaurants, but the manufacturer will ship twelve 12-ounce jars at a very reasonable price. Contact: (800) 486-2867.

romaine lettuce, and use this mixture as a flavorful fiber-rich topping for sandwiches.

NONFAT COOKING SPRAYS

Not all nonstick sprays are created equal. Some are based on artery-clogging tropical or partially hydrogenated oils, while others contain 20 percent grain alcohol which imparts a strange, "chemical" taste to food. A few have preservatives. As with all processed foods, read the label.

Nonstick sprays are another prime example of where a manufacturer's listed serving size is totally absurd. While most companies state a serving is a one-third of a second spray, I have seen products that list a spray time of one-sixteenth of a second. Maybe I'm missing something here, but for the life of me I can't figure out how to clock either of these times.

A realistic spray time is one second, which delivers one gram of fat. This amount coats a nine-inch pan, and reduces the oil to one-tenth the amount you would use if you poured it into the pan. That translates to nine grams of fat you didn't eat.

Grain alcohol is added to nonstick sprays to clarify the oil. Although it's more difficult to detect its chemical taste when used for cooking (it burns off), you will taste it if it's sprayed on cooked foods, such as popped fat-free microwave popcorn.

Tryson House Flavor Sprays are unique. These products not only prevent food from sticking, they can flavor it. You can use nonstick flavor sprays in several ways: as a quick marinade before grilling or roasting, to prevent food from sticking while frying or sautéing, or after cooking as a subtle seasoning.

Buttery Delite has a light, butter flavor that picks up the taste of steamed veggies. Try Garlic Mist as a seasoning oil for seafood and kabobs. The oregano and basil flavors make Italian Mist a natural for grilled or steamed veggies. Impart a smoky flavor to poultry and meat with Mesquite Mist. The combination of three oils in Oriental Mist makes it ideal for Asian stir-fry dishes. Although the predominant oil is peanut (its high flashpoint stands up to the intense heat used in wok cooking), it's the toasted sesame oil that catches your attention.

The only drawback to these products is that their *flavors* dissipate quickly. The trick to using nonstick sprays for *flavor* is to lightly spray your food *right* before you eat it. For instance, to get a more pronounced smoky flavor, spray Mesquite Mist on pierced poultry or meat till it shines (one-second spray), and allow the product to penetrate for several minutes before cooking. Follow it up with a light mist just before serving.

Some recipes need a longer spray time than one second. If you're craving butter-flavored popcorn, use a two-second spray time for one bag of popped fat-free microwave popcorn. While this will add 2 grams of fat, it's still a smarter choice than butter-flavored light microwave popcorns since you're eating trans-fat free canola oil. Substitute a two-second spray time of butter-flavored spray for the recommended 2 tablespoons of butter in packaged rice mixes for a savings of 26 grams of fat and 198 calories.

MICROWAVE POPCORN

Even light microwave popcorns are loaded with partially hydrogenated oils. Select a brand that doesn't use oil, such as Bearitos Organic Microwave Popcorn and Weight Watchers. Season with chili seasoning blends.

BREAKFAST CEREALS

Choose oats, whole grain and bran cereals. Limit cereals that use sugar (especially refined white sugar). Avoid cereals that use hydrogenated oils, salt and preservatives.

CANNED SOUPS

The major drawbacks to these products is that they are often high in salt and low in fiber. Choose a low-fat bean soup (spicy black bean soups are great) over noodle, vegetable and cream-based soups. Progresso Lentil soup and Black Bean Soup are excellent products.

PUREED GARLIC AND PUREED GINGER

You can find pureed garlic and pureed ginger in small jars in most well-stocked supermarkets. These two products are real time-savers, and work best in recipes that use liberal amounts of liquid, such as lentil stews. For best results, use at the beginning of the cooking process so the flavors have time to mellow. Look for preparations that use a minimal amount of preservatives to ensure the best flavor.

The Good, the Bad and the Ugly

Not all nonstick cooking sprays are equal—some contain trans-fats, preservatives or grain alcohol.

Product	Hydrogenated Oils	Alcohol	Preservatives
Naturally Lite			
Butter			
Garlic			
Olive		Yes	
Canola		Yes	
Baker's Release	Yes		Yes
Pam			
Cooking Spray		Yes	
Butter Flavor		Yes	
Imported Olive		Yes	
Crisco			
Cooking Spray			
Butter Flavor	Yes		
Wesson			
Butter			
Plain		Yes	
Pump		Yes	
Baker's Joy			
Bakery Spray	Yes		Yes
Mazola			
Cooking Spray			
Tryson House			
Buttery Delight			
Olive Mist			
Oriental Mist			
Italian Mist			
Mesquite Mist			
Cooking Magic			
Bakery Magic			

CHAPTER EIGHT

RESTAURANT RULES

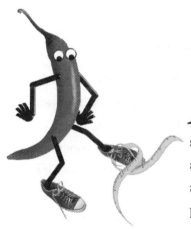

After years of eating super-sized fast foods and grande servings at restaurants, we have lost our sense of proportion. Many of us have grown accustomed to serving sizes that are more appropriate to a forklift than a fork. The problem is restaurants create their own standard portion sizes, which don't even resemble a proper serving size. Frequently, these enormous portions of food could feed a family of four.

Twenty years ago, Americans dined in restaurants twice per week. Currently, that number has jumped to eating one out of three meals out. Unfortunately, convenience has a price—your waistline. In a recent study conducted at the University of

Memphis, researchers found that women who ate out six times per week consumed 19 grams of fat and 288 calories per day more than women who ate out five times a week or less. That translates to gaining an extra 25 pounds per year! It's alarming, but not surprising!

The good news is eating out doesn't have to lead to ballooning out. The key is portion control, which is essential both for losing weight and keeping the weight off. By adopting portion-control strategies and following restaurant guidelines, you will learn new eating skills that will allow you to eat in almost any restaurant and still lose weight.

RESTAURANT GUIDELINES

- Order two large glasses of ice water with lemon. Drink one glass before your meal, and the other with your food. Better yet, substitute one glass of water with an unsweetened iced tea.
- Add crushed red pepper flakes to soups, and pickled peppers to salads. Eat these dishes at the beginning of the meal to reduce your hunger.
- Order a la carte. Although this may cost more than a price-fixed five-course meal, it gives you better control over portions so you'll be less inclined to overeat.
- Make a meal of a salad or soup, and an appetizer, which is often just the right amount of food.
- Ask your waiter to find out the weight of a fish fillet, chicken breast or the number of cups of pasta in an entree. At a deli, ask how much turkey they use in a sandwich.
- Ask the waiter if you can order appetizer portions of pasta. Many restaurants serve a four-cup portion of pasta as an entree—a serving size should be one cup.

- Request that only half of your order be brought to the table: Wrap the remainder up and take it home.
- Split a full entree with a friend.
- If you can't split the entree, eat half. Cover the remainder with salt or black pepper. The food will taste so bad, you won't be tempted to nibble at it. I've found this to be a very effective behavior modification technique.
- Ask the waiter not to bring bread and butter to your table. However, if your dining partners insist on it, move the bread and butter to the other end of the table.
- Ask for salad dressings on the side.
- Ask for sauces on the side—many sauces are high in saturated fat.
- Avoid crispy or fried foods; order broiled, grilled, roasted, baked or steamed dishes.
- Avoid cream-based sauces; order broth-based or grain-based soups.
- If you choose to have wine with your dinner, limit the portion to half a glass. Have the wine *with* your meal—you'll be inclined to overeat if you drink alcohol before the food arrives.
- If you have a favorite restaurant, choose three or four healthy, low-fat items. Automatically order one of these choices—don't even open the menu.

MAKE SUBSTITUTIONS

- Ask that dishes be prepared with a minimal amount of canola or olive oil.
- Order steamed vegetables.
- Ask that all high-fat items be eliminated—cheese, bacon, sour cream, mayonnaise, nuts, etc.

- Substitute full-fat salad dressings with salsa, lemon or lime juice, seasoned rice wine vinegar or low-fat dressings.
- Request low-fat or nonfat dairy products.

How to Make Special Requests

- Always be courteous. Select two or three dishes, and limit your questions to these items. If you interrogate the server about half the menu, he or she will lose patience. Remember, your goal is to communicate effectively.
- Make your requests clear and to the point. For instance, rather than asking if the fish is prepared with butter, tell the server, "Grill the fish dry, or use a small amount of olive oil."
- If your food comes to the table without your requests being honored, send it back!

What a Proper Portion Looks Like

One of the best ways to control the amount of food you eat is to control the amount of food that finds its way to your plate. It is crucial that you learn to recognize what a proper serving size looks like. Since you can't weigh portions in a restaurant, use these guidelines to eyeball single portions:

Food	Object
3 oz. of fish, poultry or meat	Deck of cards
1 cup of pasta	An adult fist
½ cup of rice	Half a baseball
1 cup cooked vegetables	Baseball
1-oz. slice of bread	CD case
2 tablespoons of salad dressing	Standard ice cube

BUFFETS

A smorgasbord or buffet is the ultimate challenge for someone try-ing to watch his or her waistline. Large amounts of food can tempt anyone to overeat. However, most buffets do offer a selection of foods ideally suited to the Chili Pepper Diet. Seafood, fish, roast turkey, sal-ads and fruits are among the healthiest choices.

Frequently, buffets are divided into three sections: fruits and salads, main dishes and desserts. Your best strategy for mastering the buffet is to carefully look over all the selections *before* you put food on your plate. Go back to your table, sit down, and decide which foods offer the best nutritional value for the calories. A good general guideline is to eat a large portion of fresh salad (omit high-fat items) with dress-ing on the side, followed by a small serving of seafood, fish or turkey as the entree and fresh fruit for dessert. If can't resist a high-calorie item, limit yourself to one or two bites, and eat it at the end of the meal when you're not as hungry.

Hot Hints

Recently, many restaurants have increased the size of their standard dinner plates to accommodate larger portions of food. Use salad plates for food selections instead—it's a simple, yet very effective portion-control tactic that keeps serving sizes in the right proportions.

SOUP AND SALAD BARS

Fresh salads are a good source of fiber, phytochemicals and vita-mins, but piling on the bacon bits, cheese, croutons, roasted sun-flower seeds and hard-boiled eggs defeats the purpose of choosing a salad as a healthy, low-fat meal. Moreover, a ladle of full-fat salad dressing packs close to 200 calories, so avoid making a 200-calorie salad into a 800-calorie lunch by adding 500 calories of salad dressing.

CREATING A HEALTHY SALAD

Bottom: use dark greens, such as spinach and romaine lettuce, which have a higher vitamin and nutrient content than iceberg lettuce.

Middle: fresh vegetables: bean sprouts, broccoli, cabbage, carrots, cauliflower, celery, cucumbers, green beans, jicama, mushrooms, onions, bell peppers, radishes, squash and tomatoes. Plain beans: kidney, garbanzo, etc.

Top: small amounts of shrimp, turkey or lean ham. Pickled, sliced jalapeno peppers.

*Adding pickled, sliced jalapeno peppers is crucial to making a low-fat salad taste great. No other item does a better job replacing the flavor that went out with the bacon bits, cheese and rich dressings.

Have Not

Prepared salads: coleslaw, tuna, macaroni, potato and three-bean salad, which use liberal amounts of mayonnaise, oil or sugar in their preparation.

High-fat items: cheese, bacon, avocado, croutons, roasted sunflower seeds.

Hot Hints

- If you *must* have a high-fat item, such as cheese, portion control it to a few sprinkles. It helps to think of high-fat items as "spices," not toppings. For instance, use cheese as you would black pepper.

- Limit olives to two or three. Use olives as a "spice"—not a topping. Choose Kalamata or green olives, which have more flavor than regular black olives.
- Ask the server to bring several small paper soufflé cups (2½ oz. and 1¼ oz.), such as those used for ketchup or other condiments, and use them to portion control high-fat items. For instance, if you want a taste of the New England clam chowder, fill a soufflé cup with soup. This automatically limits your portion and prevents bingeing from feeling deprived. Eat this high-fat item at the end of the meal, when you're less hungry.

High-Calorie Salad Bar Items

Condiment	Calories (per 3½ oz.)	Sodium (mg/100 gm)
Bacon bits	530	3,065
Chopped egg	160	120
Croutons	390	735
Olives, black	150	230
Olives, green	95	680
Shredded cheese (American)	380	1,125

Salad Dressings

The usual high-fat fare offered at salad bars is blue cheese, Thousand Island and Italian. Per tablespoon, these dressings pack up to eight grams of fat, and average eighty calories. Most ladles hold four to five tablespoons of dressing—you do the math. You'd be better off ordering a hamburger—with fries!

Even diet dressings can have as many as thirty to fifty calories per tablespoon, which translates to several hundred calories per ladle. Your best bet is top the salad with salsa, fresh lemon or lime juice, seasoned rice wine vinegar or balsamic vinegar (has a less acidic taste compared to red wine vinegar) mixed with a small amount of olive oil. Dress the salad at your table—not at the salad bar.

If you just *have* to eat the blue cheese dressing, limit your portion to four drops per bite. How you accomplish this daunting feat: first, dip your fork into the dressing, and then give your fork a gentle shake. This portion control technique gives you all the flavor you crave, but only a fraction of the fat.

CHINESE FOOD

Vegetables in Chinese cuisine retain both their nutrients and texture by using quick cooking methods. Unfortunately, Americanized Chinese food uses tremendous amounts of oil in the preparation of dishes. Szechwan-style dishes use even more oil than other styles of Chinese cooking. Two other pitfalls of this Asian cuisine are that it's high in sodium, usually in the form of soy sauce, and monosodium glutamate (MSG). The good news is most chefs are happy to honor your requests to use less oil, soy sauce and MSG.

Have

Wonton soup, hot-and-sour soup, steamed or stir-fried vegetables, seafood or chicken with vegetables that are steamed, boiled or lightly stir-fried, moo goo gai pan (chicken with mushrooms and vegetables), seafood or chicken prepared in a light wine or lobster sauce, steamed vegetable dumplings, velvet chicken, bean curd or tofu dishes (if not fried), Buddhist Delight, kung pao chicken (omit peanuts), steamed rice, fresh fruit, fortune cookie.

Have Not

Sizzling rice soup, coconut-based soups, egg rolls, lemon chicken, pepper steak, sweet and sour pork, Peking duck, egg foo young, moo-shu pork, oxtail, barbecued ribs, pork feet, fried shrimp, shrimp with garlic sauce, vegetable lo mein, fried wontons (fried wontons contain roughly 50 calories each), crispy noodles, fried rice, watermelon seeds, preserved eggs, Chinese sausage, eel, pork dishes, ramaki, almond cookie, green tea ice cream.

Hot Hints

- Make sure your server clearly understands your request to reduce the amount of oil, soy sauce and MSG in dishes. If there is a language problem, write it down. Ask the server to repeat the order before it is delivered to the chef.
- Ask for extra servings of red chili sauce and Chinese mustard.
- Order soup as a first course.
- Ask how tofu dishes are prepared before you order them (many chefs fry it).
- Ask that dishes be lightly stir-fried.
- Request light (sodium-reduced) soy sauce.
- Order brown rice.
- Omit nuts from dishes.

- To cut the fat in Chinese take-out food, leave the last one-half inch of food (and sauce) in the carton. You'll get all the vegetables, but avoid the oil that collects at the bottom.

AMERICAN RESTAURANTS

Fresh fish and seafood are excellent choices. They are naturally low in fat and calories, and provide an excellent source of high-quality protein. Where you run into trouble is the cooking methods. Frying and sautéing will double the calorie content of fish. Choose baked, grilled, broiled, boiled, steamed or poached dishes instead. If you must order a steak, ask that all visible fat be removed before cooking. Moreover, keep your portion size at around three ounces. Many steakhouses offer cuts of meat that weigh less than eight ounces—ask the waiter to wrap the remainder to go.

Have

Salmon, tuna, Chilean sea bass, shrimp, crab.

Turkey, chicken or lean ham sandwich on whole grain bread with double lettuce, tomato, onion, peppers and mustard.

Have Not

Avoid cream or butter sauces, fried or sautéed dishes, cream-based soups and bisques, oysters Rockefeller, club sandwiches, coleslaw, potato salad.

Hot Hints

- Order low-calorie appetizers (under 100 calories): six oysters on the half shell, melon, seafood cocktail, consommé.
- Request that small amounts of olive oil be used when grilling fish.
- Choose fresh fruit as a dessert, or limit yourself to several bites of a dining companion's rich dessert.
- Ask for a small baked potato. If the waiter brings a spud the size of a football, cut the potato in half.

JAPANESE

Japanese cuisine is naturally low in both fat and calories. Sushi is pieces of raw fish placed over a small portion of vinegared rice, secured with seaweed wrap. It is served with a spicy horseradish paste (wasabi) and pickled ginger. Depending on the type of fish used, one piece of sushi is approximately 25 to 35 calories. Sashimi consists of slices of raw fish served on a platter. Four ounces of sashimi is about 120 calories. Order chicken teriyaki, rather than beef, which is lower in both fat and calories.

Have

Miso soup, udon or noodle soup, sunumono (cucumber) salad, hijiki (seaweed) salad, wakame (seasoned seaweed) salad, chuka ika sansai (squid and mountain vegetable) salad, sushi, sashimi, edamame (boiled soy beans), chicken teriyaki, chicken sukiyaki (omit egg-based dipping sauce), steamed rice, seafood yosenabe.

Have Not

Tempura anything, eel, California roll, spicy tuna and spicy yellowtail sushi rolls if made ahead (many sushi chefs add mayonnaise to the minced fish as a binding agent), monk fish liver, pork katsu, beef negimaki.

Hot Hints

- Eat miso soup as a first course.
- Order edamame as an appetizer.
- Sushi: women—four pieces plus one roll; men six pieces plus one roll.
- Request mayonnaise and avocado not be used in the preparation of sushi rolls; substitute a small amount of chili oil in spicy tuna rolls.
- Udon soup, which contains noodles, chicken, fish cake, green onion and vegetables, is a meal in itself. Ask the waiter to bring hot pepper mix (Nanami Togarshi: chili, sesame seed, toasted seaweed, orange peel). This exceptional seasoning makes the difference between Udon soup being a good or phenomenal dish! Start with three to four shakes—it's very spicy.
- Ask for miso salad dressing on the side.
- Request light (sodium-reduced) soy sauce.
- Request MSG not be used in the preparation of dishes.
- Drink green tea—it's packed with cancer-fighting phytochemicals.

ITALIAN

Italian food can be a dieter's nightmare or delight, depending upon your choices. Simple pasta, chicken, fish and vegetables are all excellent choices. The problem arises when creamy sauces, cheese, butter and large amounts of olive oil are used in the preparation of dishes.

Have

Vegetable soup, minestrone soup, Italian salad with beans (no cheese or meat), grilled fish and seafood dishes, pasta marinara, pasta al checca, pasta arbiarrta or pasta diabalo (with hot red chilies), pasta primavera, pasta with clam sauce, gnocci (potato dumplings) with porcini mushrooms, chicken cacciatore, risotto, polenta, Italian ices, fresh fruit.

Have Not

Anything fritti (fried), antipasto salad, pasta with creamy or white sauces, pasta bolognese (meat sauce), pasta with pesto sauce, egg-plant parmigiana, veal parmigiana, lasagna, cheese-stuffed pasta (cheese tortellini or cheese ravioli), provolone cheese, mozzarella cheese, meatballs, prosciutto (Italian ham), aglio e olio (garlic and oil), tiramisu, zabaglione, gelato.

Hot Hints

- Request a side of pickled hot peppers; use as a topping on your salad.
- Request a side of crushed red pepper flakes; use as a seasoning on pasta and fish dishes.
- Order wine by the glass—not the carafe. Dilute white wine with half club soda to equal a six-ounce serving.

- If you must have cheese, use a small amount (one tablespoon) of sharp Parmesan cheese. This cheese has more flavor, and you'll be satisfied with smaller portions.
- If you just can't resist pizza, order a thin-crust pie with half the cheese and double portions of garlic, onions, bell peppers and mushrooms (no sausage, pepperoni or olives). Better yet, leave out the mozzarella cheese, and sprinkle a small amount of a sharp parmesan and lots of crushed red pepper flakes when it comes to your table. Limit your portion to two slices.

DELI

The problem with deli food is twofold: The portions tend to be enormous, and many of the items are swimming in artery-clogging saturated fats. However, you can enjoy a healthy meal if you choose wisely. Soups, fish plates, roast chicken or a turkey sandwich are among the healthier choices, and be diligent using portion-control techniques. For instance, most delis serve seven-ounce bagels, which pack five hundred calories (twenty years ago, a standard bagel was three ounces), and turkey sandwiches come with six to nine ounces of turkey—not the three ounces considered a serving.

Have

Borscht (no sour cream), matzo ball soup, chicken noodle soup, chicken and rice soup, barley soup, lentil soup, fish plate, turkey sandwich (half) with mustard and a side of onions and tomatoes, lox and bagel (half) with nonfat or low-fat cream cheese and a side of tomatoes, roast chicken (skin removed), roast turkey (skin removed), gefilte fish, kippered herring, pickled herring, kasha (buckwheat groats), pickles, pickled green tomatoes, rye bread, whole-grain bread, angel food cake with berries.

Have Not

Blintzes, sour cream, mayonnaise, cheese, pastrami, brisket, corned beef, tongue, tuna salad sandwich, gravy, potato latkes, chopped liver, flanken, potato salad, coleslaw, grebnes (cracklings), smaltz (chicken fat), salami, bubke (coffee cake), kuchen (cake), lakach (honey cake), sour cream herring, rugalah (strudel), hamentaschen (cookies), mandel bread, cheesecake.

Hot Hints

- Ask for a side of pickled peppers with a sandwich.
- When you order a sandwich, ask for a side of tomatoes, cucumbers and onions. They add both moisture and flavor.
- Substitute fresh fruit for potato salad and coleslaw.
- Substitute mustard for mayonnaise on sandwiches. This will cut 200 to 300 calories and 20 to 30 grams of fat.
- Ask for whole-grain bread or pita bread, which have more fiber than white bread or rolls. Order a water bagel; limit your portion to half a bagel. Pass on the sesame and poppy seed bagels—the seeds can add up to 4 grams of fat.
- Order sandwiches without cheese. If you must have cheese, use a quarter of a slice.

MEXICAN

American-style Mexican food tends to be high in fat, but you can easily transform this cuisine into healthier meals by leaving out the cheese, sour cream, guacamole and refried beans. Steer clear of fried food, beef and pork dishes. Fish, chicken, corn-based dishes, salsas, boiled beans and plain tortillas are all excellent, lower-calorie choices. As for the tortilla chips, ask the waiter to bring soft corn tortillas with the salsa instead. Fried tortilla chips are fifteen calories per chip, and several handfuls add up to three hundred calories in no time.

Have

Black bean soup, tortilla soup (omit cheese and fried tortilla strips), gazapacho, Yucatan lime soup, salsas, corn tortillas, beans in broth (boiled beans with chilies), soft tacos with a chicken or grilled fish filling, Mexican salad plate, nopales (catus) salad, jicama salad, steamed chayote (Mexican squash), boiled calabazita (squash), arroz con pollo (rice with chicken), vegetarian burrito (beans, rice, lettuce, onions, tomatoes, cilantro, salsa), grilled chicken or fish, pescado Veracruzana (fish in a Veracruz sauce consisting of olive oil, onions, green olives and capers), toasted with either boiled beans and rice or stewed chicken filling; hold the cheese, sour cream and guacamole. Do not eat the fried flour tortilla shell—think of it as the plate.

Have Not

Mexican sausage (chorizo), beef or pork dishes, guacamole, sofrito, refried beans, tamales, mole dishes, cheese, sour cream, chili rellenos, corn fritter, cheese enchiladas, flauta (rolled, stuffed and fried tortillas), taquitos and flan.

Hot Hints

- Substitute soft corn tortilla for flour tortillas (flour tortillas use lard or partially hydrogenated oil in their preparation).
- Ask the server to bring several bowls of different salsas; use salsa as a salad dressing, topping for soft tacos, tostadas. etc. Make it clear to the waiter that you want one-cup servings of salsa—not a soufflé-cup serving.
- Request a side of pickled jalapenos, or fresh chopped chilies with your order.
- Substitute high-fat items (cheese, sour cream, guacamole) with double portions of tomatoes, cilantro and onions.
- If you must have cheese, use small amounts of a sharp Mexican cheese, such as cotija. Although it is not lower in fat than cheddar or jack cheese, it has more flavor so you'll be satisfied with less. (One tablespoon of cotija has two grams of total fat and one gram of saturated fat.)

CARIBBEAN

Fiery peppers, spicy rubs, ginger, lime, mango, coconut, seafood and root vegetables are the signature flavors of this exhilarating tropical cuisine. Your best bets are jerk dishes, which are seasoned with hot peppers, onions and spices; then smoked.

Unfortunately, many dishes feature ingredients that are high in saturated fat—salt pork, coconut milk and butter. Although rice and beans (or rice and peas) sounds healthy, this dish incorporates liberal amounts of coconut milk. Steer clear of callaloo (one-pot) dishes, which contain both salt pork and coconut milk.

Have

Jerk chicken, grilled seafood or fish, ackee and saltfish (omit salt pork).

Have Not

Dishes using coconut milk, salt pork, bacon, ham hock or butter in their preparation, pork dishes, callaloos, rice and beans, fried plantains, cornmeal pudding, sweet potato pone, coconut.

Hot Hints

- Ask your waiter which dishes contain coconut milk, salt pork, bacon, ham hock or butter.
- Escoveitch fish is lightly pan-fried, then cooked with onions, bell peppers and vinegar. Request small amounts of oil be used in its preparation; add hot peppers.
- Substitute fresh tropical fruits topped with fresh lime juice for rich desserts.

THAI

This vibrant Asian cuisine is perfumed with spicy, sweet, sour and aromatic flavors. Lemongrass, chili, curry, coconut, lime, basil and peanut are the ingredients that define Thai food. Order seafood, fish, chicken, soup and noodle dishes prepared with chilies, lime juice and basil. Avoid entrees featuring coconut milk and nuts. Steer clear of pad Thai (this noodle dish uses liberal amounts of oil, peanuts and egg in its preparation), pork dishes and fried appetizers. Also, go easy on the satay (peanut sauce) that accompanies many grilled dishes.

Have

Gai yang (grilled chicken served over cabbage with a virtually fat-free sweet chili sauce), poy sain (seafood sautéed with mushrooms, onions, bamboo shoots and string beans), Thai chicken (omit nuts), larb, mango salsa, papaya salad (omit peanuts), tom yum kung.

Have Not

Tom kha kai, meekrob, Thai sausage salad, pork dishes, egg rolls, fried shrimp, fried rice dishes, curries, pad Thai.

Hot Hints

- Request vegetable oil be used in the preparation of dishes, rather than lard or coconut oil.
- Pass on nam prik (spicy peanut sauce) and soa nam (which contains coconut); both are loaded with fat.

INDIAN

Although Indian cuisine appears to be healthy—it's spicy, based on complex carbohydrates (garbanzo beans and lentils) and uses lots of vegetables—many dishes are loaded with fat. Appetizers and breads are deep-fried, while vegetables and meat are sautéed in ghee (clarified butter). Your best bet is to stick with dishes that are marinated and roasted in a tandoori (clay) oven, and avoid entrees that list ghee, coconut, nuts or cream sauces in the menu.

Have

Mulligataway soup, chicken, fish or shrimp tika, raita, mint chutney, naan, chapati, dal (without cream), masala (small amount of oil), chicken vindaloo (spicy tomato-based sauce; no cream).

Have Not

Samosas, koftas, dosa and pakoras (deep-fried appetizers), poori (deep-fried bread), dishes described as biryani, korma, mali (contain liberal amounts of oil or cream), meat dishes, Indian desserts.

FAST FOODS

Although fast foods won't make the Nutrition Hall of Fame, you can maneuver your way into a healthier meal by following three cardinal rules: no fried food, order it "plain," and don't "super-size." The obvious culprits to avoid are fried chicken, burgers and fries. However, looks can be deceiving. One of the fattiest fast foods you can eat is a taco salad at Taco Bell. Far from being a healthy alternative, it packs 52 grams of fat and a whopping 850 calories. This diet disaster is in the same ballpark as a double bacon cheeseburger. The worst product in fast-food land is Taco Bell's Mucho Grande Nachos. A mountain of grease masquerading as a side dish, it contains 82 grams of artery-clogging fat, and weighs in at 1,350 calories!

Many fast-food junkies are under the false impression that fish and chicken dishes are lower in fat and calories than burgers. In truth, most are not. Chicken and fish sandwiches are usually battered, then fried. The creamy "secret sauce" adds another heart-stopping 13 grams of fat. To put things in perspective, the Chicken Supreme Sandwich at Jack in the Box contains 39 grams of fat and 641 calories; the Fish

Supreme sandwich packs 27 grams of fat and 510 calories. A cheese-burger has 14 grams of fat, and 315 calories!

A better choice is ordering a fish or chicken sandwich that is grilled, baked or roasted. Order the sandwich "plain," which translates in fast foodese to "leave out the mayonnaise sauce," and be sure to hold the cheese.

Beverages

In the United States, over $49 billion a year is spent on soda alone—that's more than the gross domestic product of Ireland! Currently, Americans drink 56 gallons of soda per year—that translates to nearly 600 twelve-ounce cans of soda per person! It's alarming, but not surprising.

Over the last two decades, the average American has increased their sugar consumption from 10 pounds per year to over 21 pounds per year. This dramatic increase has been linked to "super-sized" sodas. For instance, the 7-Eleven Gulp was no longer big enough for many Americans, so this convenience store chain introduced their runaway hit—the Double Gulp. To put this in perspective, one twelve-ounce can of soda contains 10 teaspoons of sugar. A Double Gulp Coke holds over 53 teaspoons of sugar! This is not a beverage—it's "liquid candy."

A 7-Eleven Double Gulp (64 ounce) Coke contains an astonishing 792 calories! Ordering a jumbo Diet Coke may not be healthier choice either—especially if you're a women. While the scientific data on the detrimental effects of artificial sweeteners remains unclear, Diet Coke also contains phosphoric acid, which leeches calcium. This may increase your risk for osteoporosis (brittle bones). Don't make a 64-ounce Diet Coke a daily habit. Order the 32-ounce size instead.

Your best bet is to order an unsweetened iced tea. It's the one fast-food item you can "super-size" without regret. Although tea contains caffeine, it is a better choice than a Diet Coke. Better yet, order a medium iced tea and a large water.

(Nonfat milk is also a good alternative, but many fast-food franchises don't carry it.)

Diet Soda Beverages

Containing Phosphoric Acid	Without Phosphoric Acid
Diet Coke	Diet Sprite
Diet Pepsi	Diet 7-Up
Diet Dr Pepper	Diet A&W Cream
R.C. Diet Rite	Diet Vernor's (Ginger soda)
	Diet Cherry 7-Up
	Diet Mountain Dew
	Diet Sunkist

Healthier Choices at Fast-Food Restaurants

Franchise/Product	Calories	Fat (g)	Protein (g)
McDonald's			
Chicken McGrill (plain without mayo)	340	7	26
Grilled Chicken Caesar Salad			
(fat-free herb vinaigrette)	100	2.5	17
Regular hamburger (plain; substitute			
mustard or ketchup)	280	10	12
*Order with double onion, tomato, lettuce.			
Sauces (Avoid—contain fat)			
Honey Mustard	60	3.5	0
Hot Mustard	45	4.5	0
Jack in the Box			
Chicken Fajita Pita (without the			
American cheese)	235	5	20
*Request double onion, tomato and lettuce.			
Burger King			
Chicken Broiler Sandwich (plain)	390	8	29
*Order with double onion, tomato, lettuce.			
Use ketchup and mustard—sandwich is dry;			
Use ketchup over tomatoes; mustard on the chicken.			
Sauces			
(Avoid—contain fat)			
Honey Mustard Dipping Sauce	90	6	0
Wendy's			
Grilled Chicken Salad (with fat-free			
French dressing)	235	8	22
Grilled Chicken Sandwich (plain)	300	8	24
*Order with double onion, tomato, lettuce.			
Use ketchup and mustard—sandwich is dry:			
Use ketchup over tomatoes; mustard on the chicken.			
Taco Bell			
Soft Taco–steak (without cheddar cheese)	160	5	12
*Order 2 tacos (with extra tomato, onion)			
Soft Taco–chicken (without cheddar cheese)	160	5	11
*Order 2 tacos (with extra tomato, onion)			

Healthier Choices at Fast-Food Restaurants

Franchise/Product	Calories	Fat (g)	Protein (g)
Taco Bell (cont'd)			
Sauces			
Green Sauce (hotter than Red Sauce)	5	0	0
Border Hot (has better flavor than Border Fire)	0	0	0
Fiesta Salsa		0	0
Southwest Salsa	20	0	0
El Pollo Loco			
Tostada Salad (without shell & sour cream)	304	11	30
Numbers will be lower without cheese			
*Add onions, cilantro and 4–5 ladles of hot salsa.			
Taco Al Carbon	164	6	13
Pinto Beans	185	4	15
Make-your-own soft taco (2)			
Corn tortilla			
4.5-inch	32	0.5	1
6-inch	70	1	1
Flame-Broiled Chicken Breast	160	6	26
*Add 4–5 ladles of hot chipotle or pico de gallo salsa.			
Koo Koo Roo			
4 oz. White Turkey Meat Sandwich	153	1	34
with one of the following:			
12-Vegetable Chopped Salad	78	1	5
(with ½ serving of chopped salad dressing)			
Cucumber Salad	30	0	0
Koo Koo Roo Slaw	55	2	1
Tangy Tomato Salad	56	3	1
Tomato Basil Pasta	108	2	3
Ten Vegetable Soup	121	3	3
Chicken Chili Soup	98	2	8
Turkey Dumpling Soup	166	4	19
Lentil Salad	175	5	11
with lahvash (flatbread)	94	0	4

Healthier Choices at Fast-Food Restaurants

Franchise/Product	Calories	Fat (g)	Protein (g)
Subway			
(6-inch sub on whole wheat)			
Order with double onion, tomato, bell peppers,			
jalapenos, oregano, salt and pepper.			
*Use Dijon mustard as a condiment—sandwich is dry.			
Turkey (without cheese and mayo)	254	3.5	16
Ham (without cheese and mayo)	261	4.5	17
Roast Beef (without cheese and mayo)	264	4.5	18
Roasted Chicken Breast (without cheese and mayo)	348	6.0	27

SPECIAL OCCASIONS

Never go to a party hungry—you'll be inclined to overeat. Your best bet to prevent bingeing is to eat a small meal before you go. A few suggestions you might try are a soup or salad containing chilies and a small serving of lean protein; half a turkey sandwich with chilies, lettuce, tomatoes and onions; or a half a bagel with nonfat cream cheese spread.

Another strategy that prevents overeating is to formulate a plan before you leave that sets guidelines for both food and alcohol. For instance, decide in advance to limit your alcoholic beverages to one or two wine spritzers (no more than six ounces of alcohol), and alternate with a club soda between drinks. Your best bet in the hors d'oeuvres department is a chilled seafood (clams, shrimp, oysters) and fresh vegetables. Be sure to limit yourself to a handful of each. If you choose to eat rich hors d'oeuvres, limit yourself to one serving of each.

Other tactics for controlling your appetite include: arriving at the party a little late, delaying drinking until fifteen minutes after you have arrived, waiting thirty minutes before eating hors d'oeuvres, positioning yourself a good distance from the buffet table and leaving after several hours.

VACATIONS

The secret for not gaining weight on vacations is planning. When you purchase your airline ticket, order a low-fat meal and a fruit plate. Be sure to pack a supply of chilies. However, it's a good idea to check with your carrier about possible restrictions. Once you have arrived at your destination, select one meal per day that you can indulge a little more than at other meals—breakfast or lunch is best because your metabolism is naturally revving in a higher gear.

When you're traveling, it's important to balance your nutrition. In other words, select meals in relation to what else you will be eating during the day. For instance, if you have a heavy lunch, dinner should be light. If you eat lox for breakfast and shrimp for lunch, choose a dinner that has less protein and more complex carbohydrates.

If you choose to drink alcohol on your vacation, make trade-offs. For instance, if you drink a wine spritzer at dinner, forgo a serving of bread, rice, pasta or potato from one of your daily meals. One three-ounce glass of wine translates to dropping one starch. One six-ounce glass of wine equals one serving of starch and half a serving of fruit. Also, do not exceed one drink per day, and limit your alcohol intake to two drinks per week.

6757058862

READER/CUSTOMER CARE SURVEY

We care about your opinions. Please take a moment to fill out this Reader Survey card and mail it back to us. As a special **"thank you"** we'll send you exciting news about interesting books and a valuable **Gift Certificate**

Please PRINT using ALL CAPITALS

Name First [_____] MI.[__] Last Name [_____]

Address [_____]

City [_____] ST [__] Zip [_____]

Phone # ([____]) [____] - [____] Fax # ([____]) [____] - [____]

Email [_____]

BA1

(1) Gender:
○ Female
○ Male

(2) Age:
○ 13-19 ○ 40-49
○ 20-29 ○ 50-59
○ 30-39 ○ 60+

(3) Your children's age(s):
Please fill in all that apply.
○ 6 or Under ○ 15-18
○ 7-10 ○ 19+
○ 11-14

(8) Marital Status:
○ Married
○ Single
○ Divorced / Widowed

(9) Was this book:
○ Purchased For Yourself?
○ Received As a Gift?

(10)How many HCI books have you bought or read?
○ 1 ○ 3
○ 2 ○ 4+

(11) Did this book meet your expectations?
○ Yes
○ No

(12) How did you find out about this book? *Please fill in ONE.*
○ Personal Recommendation
○ Store Display
○ TV/Radio Program
○ Bestseller List
○ Website
○ Advertisement/Article or Book
○ Catalog or Mailing
○ Other _____

(13) What FIVE subject areas do you enjoy reading about most? *Rank only FIVE. Choose 1 for your favorite, 2 for second favorite, etc.*

	1	2	3	4	5
Self Development	○	○	○	○	○
Parenting	○	○	○	○	○
Spirituality/Inspiration	○	○	○	○	○
Family and Relationships	○	○	○	○	○
Health and Nutrition	○	○	○	○	○
Recovery	○	○	○	○	○
Business/Professional	○	○	○	○	○
Entertainment	○	○	○	○	○
Sports	○	○	○	○	○
Teen Issues	○	○	○	○	○
Pets	○	○	○	○	○

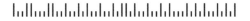
FOLD HERE

BA1

9396058864

(25) Are you:
○ A Parent?
○ A Grandparent

(18) Where do you purchase most of your books?
Please fill in your top TWO choices only.
○ General Bookstore
○ Religious Bookstore
○ Warehouse / Price Club
○ Discount or Other Retail Store
○ Website
○ Book Club / Mail Order

(20) What type(s) of magazines do you SUBSCRIBE to?
Fill in up to FIVE categories.
○ Parenting
○ Sports
○ Fashion
○ Business / Professional
○ World News / Current Events
○ General Entertainment
○ Homemaking, Cooking, Crafts
○ Women's Issues
○ Other (please specify) _____

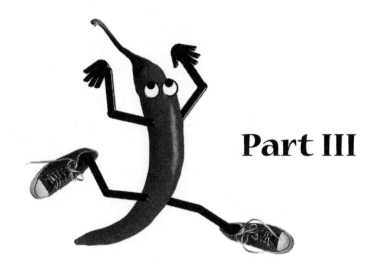

Part III

THE CHILI PEPPER DIET RECIPES FOR SUCCESS

CHAPTER NINE

HOT AND HEALTHY RECIPES

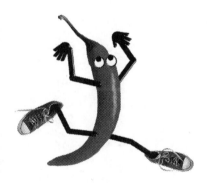

BREADSPREADS

SPICY DIJON SPREAD

Makes: 18 servings

According to researchers, the largest sources of fat in American women's diets are margarine and mayonnaise. I use commercial low-fat or nonfat mayonnaise as a base, and add chilies, herbs or salsas to create my own delicious "breadspreads" for sandwiches. This recipe is fabulous on a turkey sandwich!

½ cup nonfat mayonnaise *a scant ⅛ cup water*
¼ cup Dijon mustard *4 pickled pepperoncini peppers*

1. Put all ingredients in a blender. Puree until smooth.

*Kept refrigerated, this will last a week or more.

Serving size: 1 tablespoon

CAL	FAT	PROT	CARB	FIBER	SODIUM
9	0.1 gm	0.0 gm	1.4+ gm	0.1+ gm	187 mg

OLIVE CREAM CHEESE SPREAD

Makes: 7 servings

1 (8 oz.) container of nonfat cream cheese, softened to room temperature
20 small green olives stuffed with pimento, minced
¼ teaspoon juice from olives

1. In a small bowl, whip cream cheese with a fork until creamy.

2. Mix together the cream cheese, capers and caper juice.

3. Chill for 24 hours.

*Kept refrigerated, this will last a week or more.

Serving size: 2 tablespoons

CAL	FAT	PROT	CARB	FIBER	SODIUM
27	0.4 gm	3.4 gm	1.8 gm	0.0+ gm	241 mg

TIP: The easiest way to mince the olives is with a hand chopper.

Caper Cream Cheese Spread

Makes: 7 servings

1 (8 oz.) container of nonfat cream cheese, softened to room temperature
1 heaping tablespoon capers
¼ teaspoon juice from capers

1. In a small bowl, whip cream cheese with a fork until creamy.

2. Mix together the cream cheese, capers and caper juice with a fork.

3. Chill for 24 hours.

Kept refrigerated, this will last a week or more.

Serving size: 2 tablespoons

CAL	FAT	PROT	CARB	FIBER	SODIUM
26	0.0 gm	4.4 gm	1.7 gm	0.1 gm	211 mg

CHEF JAMIE SHANNON'S CHIPOTLE KETCHUP

Makes: 35 servings

4 chipotle chilies, rehydrated in 3 oz. cold water
1 head of roasted garlic
1½ tablespoon of olive oil
3 oz. corn syrup
½ oz. rice wine vinegar

1. Rehydrate chilies until soft (12 hours overnight).

2. In oven, roast one head of peeled garlic and 4 red bell peppers, lightly coated with olive oil and season with salt and pepper at 350 degrees for 20 minutes or until garlic is brown or peppers blister. If garlic is dark and peppers are not quite done, remove and continue to roast peppers.

3. When peppers are blistered or dark, put in stainless steel bowl with drippings and cover with plastic wrap. Let cool.

4. After peppers have cooled, peel and seed. Put back in liquid that remains in bowl.

5. Take rehydrated chilies and liquid and place in food processor with roasted garlic and roasted red peppers and blend.

6. Slowly add corn syrup and vinegar. Let blend until all is mixed. Taste and adjust seasoning with salt and pepper.

*Kept refrigerated, this will last a week or more.

Serving size: 1 tablespoon

CAL	FAT	PROT	CARB	FIBER	SODIUM
13	0 gm	0.2 gm	3.2 gm	0.2+ gm	17 mg

SAVORY POULTRY BREADSPREADS

Makes: 4 servings

Adding a dry recado to low-fat mayonnaise is a wonderful way to impart robust, smoky flavors to a bland turkey or chicken sandwich. Don't worry if the recado has lumps (mixtures of garlic, chilies and herbs)—they translate into savory bursts of flavor in the sandwich.

½ cup low-fat mayonnaise
1 heaping teaspoon of Chili Pepper Diet Recado (dry) seasoning
(see recipe under Seasoning Blends)

1. Add Chili Pepper Diet Recado to low-fat mayonnaise.
2. Chill overnight to allow the flavors to meld.

*Kept refrigerated, this will last a week or more.

Serving size: 2 tablespoons

CAL	FAT	PROT	CARB	FIBER	SODIUM
31	2.0 gm	0 gm	4.2 gm	0 gm	281 mg

EGG DISHES

EGGS WITH MUSHROOMS, ONIONS AND BROCCOLI

Makes: 1 serving

A little olive oil goes a long way to bring out the flavor of broccoli. This recipe uses a "steam-fry" technique, which allows you to significantly reduce the amount of oil traditionally used for sautéing these rather dry vegetables.

> 1 teaspoon olive oil
> ¾ cup broccoli florets, chopped
> 1–2 serrano (or red jalapeno) chilies, minced
> 1 tablespoon chopped onion
> 2 small mushrooms, ¼-inch slice
> 1 teaspoon water
> 4 egg whites, scrambled
> dash of kosher salt and black pepper

1. Heat an 8-inch nonstick pan on medium heat until hot.

2. Add 1 tsp. olive oil and heat until thin. Tilt pan and allow heated oil to cover the entire bottom surface of the pan. Pour off ½ the amount of oil—about ½ teaspoon should remain in pan.

3. Add broccoli and chilies. Stir-fry until the broccoli changes color to a bright green.

4. Add onions, mushrooms and water and stir. Reduce heat to medium-low and cover pan with lid. Allow vegetables to steam until tender. Remove lid and stir until water evaporates.

5. Add egg whites and cook until set. Salt and pepper to taste.

CAL	FAT	PROT	CARB	FIBER	SODIUM
129	2.8 gm	18.1 gm	9.5 gm	4.0 gm	242 mg

THREE-PEPPER OMELET

Makes: 1 serving

Chefs mix green and red chilies to get a balance of flavors. In this dish, the poblano chili imparts a smoky, fruity taste; the serrano chili adds heat; and the red bell pepper lends sweetness, which gives the omelet complexity and depth. Also, there is a nutritional reason for mixing red and green peppers in dishes— the green chili provides vitamin C and the red bell pepper supplies vitamin A (antioxidants that provide protection from cancer).

1 large poblano chili, roasted, peeled and sliced (½ cup)
2 tablespoons red bell pepper, diced (about ¼ large red bell pepper)
1 serrano pepper, diced (remove seeds if you are not used to chilies)
2 tablespoons onion, diced (about ¼ medium white onion)
1 egg plus 3 egg whites, scrambled
1 tablespoon minced cilantro
kosher salt and pepper to taste

1. Preheat an 8-inch nonstick pan on medium-low heat and spray with olive oil nonstick spray (one-second spray).

2. Add chilies, bell pepper and onions and stir. Cover, and cook until tender. Remove from pan and wipe pan clean.

3. Heat 8-inch nonstick pan on medium-low heat until hot. Spray with olive oil spray (two-second spray). Add egg mixture. As egg starts to set, pull one corner of egg mixture toward the center of the pan and tilt pan to allow uncooked egg to cover. Repeat with other three corners. Cook until set.

4. Top with vegetable mixture and cilantro.

5. Salt and pepper to taste.

6. Fold over and serve.

CAL	FAT	PROT	CARB	FIBER	SODIUM
157	4.6 gm	17.2 gm	11.6 gm	2.2 gm	512 mg

BREAKFAST BURRITO

Makes: 1 serving

½ cup chopped onion (about ½ small yellow onion)
2 seranno chilies, minced
1 large roma tomato, chopped (about ½ cup)
1 whole egg plus 2 whites, scrambled
½ slice Kraft 2% Milk Fat Cheese
1 8-inch low-fat flour tortilla
1 tablespoon minced cilantro

1. Heat an 8-inch nonstick pan on medium-low heat until hot.

2. Spray with butter-flavored nonstick spray (one-second spray).

3. Add onions and serrano chillies, cover, and cook till translucent.

4. Increase heat to medium-high. Add tomato and move vegetable mixture around in pan with spatula to evaporate liquid.

5. Reduce heat to medium-low. Add eggs and stir until set.

6. Place cheese over eggs, turn off heat and cover pan with lid until cheese is melted.

7. Dampen hands with water and rub over both sides of tortilla to moisten it.

8. Heat a 10-inch nonstick pan on medium heat.

9. Place damp tortilla in preheated pan and cook until soft.

10. Spoon egg mixture over bottom third of tortilla and top with cilantro. Fold in ends of tortilla and roll up.

CAL	FAT	PROT	CARB	FIBER	SODIUM
333	6.8 gm	21.9 gm	46.7 gm	5.9 gm	744 mg

TIP: You can heat a dry flour tortilla (wrapped in plastic) in a microwave for 30 seconds between plastic wrap. However, the microwave often changes the texture of the tortilla and makes it "gummy."

VEGETARIAN DISHES

VEGETARIAN BURRITO

Makes: 1 serving

⅓ cup pre-cooked Rice Verde (see recipe) (can substitute brown rice)
½ cup canned pinto beans, drained
1 8-inch low-fat flour tortilla
1 tablespoon of feta or cotija cheese
1 tablespoon of minced white onion mixed with 1 tablespoon of minced
   cilantro
¼ cup fresh salsa of choice
1 small roma tomato, chopped
1 pickled jalapeno
shredded lettuce

1. Heat rice and beans in a microwave until warm.

2. Dampen hands with water and rub over both sides of tortilla to moisten it
   (water softens low-fat tortilla).

3. Heat a 10-inch nonstick pan on medium heat.

4. Place damp tortilla in preheated pan and cook until soft. Remove tortilla and
   place on plate.

5. Spoon rice mixture over bottom third of tortilla. Top with beans, rice, cheese,
   cilantro and onion mixture, salsa, tomato, jalapeno and lettuce.

6. Fold in ends of tortilla and roll up.

CAL	FAT	PROT	CARB	FIBER	SODIUM
385	3.9 gm	15.7 gm	65.3 gm	10.8 gm	1,147 mg

TIP: Rinsing the beans will reduce their sodium content by one-third.

ROASTED POBLANO HUMMUS

Makes: 2 servings

Many people shy away from beans because they taste bland. To make these healthy legumes more palatable, either lots of fat or hefty doses of sugar are used to pick up the flavor. The secret to the success of this dish is fire-roasted chilies, which supply not only taste but texture. It's crucial to roast the poblano peppers directly over a gas flame (creates a more concentrated smoky taste than broiling)—their smoky flavor enhances the smoky, sweet taste of the morita chilies. Pair this dish with pita bread for a nutritious vegetarian meal.

1 15-ounce can garbanzo beans
2 cloves garlic, chopped
⅛ teaspoon kosher salt
⅓ cup chopped cilantro
1 cup chopped roasted, peeled and seeded poblano pepper
    (1 very large or 2 medium poblanos)
1 tablespoon brine from pickled jalapenos
1 teaspoon ground cumin
1 teaspoon olive oil

1. Drain garbanzo beans and reserve juice.
2. Put garlic and salt in a mortar and crush to a paste.
3. Put cilantro and garlic mixture in a blender and blend for several seconds until smooth.
4. Add roasted poblano peppers and blend to a smooth paste.
5. Add garbanzo beans, jalapeno brine, cumin and olive oil to vegetable mixture, and blend to a smooth, creamy consistency. Add 1–2 tablespoons of reserved bean juice if mixture is too thick, and blend again.
6. Chill for 24 hours to let flavors "marry."

Kept refrigerated, this will last for five days.

Serving size: 1 cup

CAL	FAT	PROT	CARB	FIBER	SODIUM
177	4.6 gm	7.5 gm	28.4 gm	6.9 gm	699 gm

With ½ pita bread

CAL	FAT	PROT	CARB	FIBER	SODIUM
272	5.6 gm	11.0 gm	46.4 gm	8.4 gm	889 mg

ROASTED RED PEPPER
AND BASIL HUMMUS

Makes: 2 servings

This recipe is a low-fat version of the classic Middle Eastern dish, hummus. The secret to the success of this dish is roasting the bell peppers directly over a gas flame to create a rich, smoky flavor. Blending the beans and caramelized vegetables in stages creates the creamy texture traditionally supplied by the high-fat sesame seed paste, tahina. Marinating the beans in lemon juice enhances the lemon taste—the perfect counterpoint flavor to balance the salty taste of the capers. Pair this dish with pita bread for a nutritious vegetarian meal.

> 1 15-ounce can garbanzo beans
> ½ cup fresh lemon juice
> 4 morita chilies (can substitute 1 canned chipotle chili in sauce)
> 2 cloves garlic, minced
> ⅛ teaspoon kosher salt
> 2 red bell peppers, roasted, peeled and seeded (1 cup chopped)
> 1 tablespoon brine from Kalamata olives
> 1 tablespoon fresh lemon juice
> 1–2 tablespoons of canned bean juice
> 1 teaspoon olive oil
> 4 Kalamata olives, cured in brine (not oil)
> ⅓ cup chopped basil, plus 2 tablespoons of slivered basil
> 1 tablespoon capers, drained

1. Drain garbanzo beans and reserve juice. Marinate beans in lemon juice for 30 minutes.

2. Rehydrate morita chilies (whole) in water for 30 minutes if dry. Slice chilies into slivers.

3. Put garlic and salt in a mortar and crush to a paste.

4. Put chopped basil with garlic-salt mixture in a blender and blend into a smooth paste.

5. Add roasted bell peppers, chilies, lemon juice, olives and olive oil to basil-garlic paste in blender and blend to a smooth paste.

6. Add beans, brine and bean juice to vegetable mixture, and blend on pulse setting of blender to achieve a smooth, creamy consistency (you will have to pulse and stir several times). Add more bean or lemon juice if mixture is too thick. Remove bean mixture to another dish.

7. Add capers and slivered basil, fold into bean mixture and stir. Chill for 24 hours to let flavors "marry."

Kept refrigerated, this will last for five days.

Serving size: 1 cup

CAL	FAT	PROT	CARB	FIBER	SODIUM
188	5.5 gm	7.3 gm	29.4 gm	7.3+ gm	834 mg

with ½ pita bread

CAL	FAT	PROT	CARB	FIBER	SODIUM
283	6.5 gm	10.8 gm	47.4 gm	8.8 gm	1,024 mg

GOAT CHEESE PIZZA WITH OLIVES

Makes: 1 serving

Pizza is one of those foods we love—and crave. Unfortunately, many of the frozen pies on the market don't measure up for a low-fat diet—both in taste and nutrition. This recipe raises the bar for low-fat pizza: it uses fresh (not frozen) Armenian pizza bread as a base and you add the toppings! Just be sure to accurately measure out the goat cheese to keep the fat grams low. You can find Armenian pizza bread (Spicy Onion and Tomato, Vegetable and Spicy Spinach) in the bread section of Costco, Whole Foods Market or in Middle Eastern markets.

1 Middle Eastern style low-fat thin-crust spicy spinach pizza
⅓ cup Friendship Spreadable (1% Milkfat) Whipped Low-Fat Cottage
  Cheese
3 pitted Kalamata olives, chopped
½ ounce goat cheese, crumbled
1 teaspoon red pepper flakes

1. Preheat toaster oven to 450°.
2. With a knife, spread cottage cheese over pizza crust and top with goat cheese.
3. Place chopped olives over cheeses, and sprinkle with crushed red pepper flakes.
4. Place pizza on a baking sheet and cook for 10 minutes, or until cheese melts.

CAL	FAT	PROT	CARB	FIBER	SODIUM
252	7.2 gm	18.3 gm	30.3 gm	2.7+ gm	855 mg

Oatmeal with Cinnamon and Blueberries

Makes: 1 serving

In this recipe, blueberries are paired with cinnamon to enhance the health-promoting properties of oatmeal. Blueberries contain powerful antioxidants that prevent urinary tract infections and reduce memory loss. Cinnamon improves the body's sensitivity (responsiveness) to insulin. Moreover, cinnamon's spicy, sweet note balances the tartness of the berries, creating a seductively rich, fruity flavor. A nice change from the traditional raisin rendition!

⅔ cup instant oatmeal
1⅓ cups water
½ teaspoon of cinnamon
¼ cup dried blueberries (can substitute raisins)
dash of kosher salt
½ cup of nonfat milk

1. In medium bowl, add ⅔ cup oatmeal and 1⅓ cups of water.

2. Stir and place in microwave oven (do not cover). Heat for 1–2 minutes.

3. Add cinnamon, a dash of kosher salt and stir.

4. Sprinkle blueberries over oatmeal mixture.

5. Top with ½ cup of nonfat milk.

CAL	FAT	PROT	CARB	FIBER	SODIUM
250	3 gm	11 gm	47 gm	7 gm	73 mg

CREAM OF WHEAT

Makes: 1 serving

For some "carboholics," a warm bowl of Cream of Wheat is the ultimate comfort food—they just love its rich and creamy texture. However, you'll be hungry within an hour unless it's prepared with an ample serving of nonfat milk. Also, milk does a much better job than water to enhance the creamy texture of the wheat.

1 cup nonfat milk
1 tablespoon nonfat milk powder
⅛ teaspoon kosher salt
3 tablespoons Cream of Wheat

1. Put milk, milk powder, salt and Cream of Wheat into a bowl.
2. Heat in microwave oven on high for 1 minute and stir.
3. Reheat in microwave oven for 30 seconds and stir. Reheat for another 30 seconds or until thick.

CAL	FAT	PROT	CARB	FIBER	SODIUM
289	1.2 gm	19.9 gm	48.4 gm	1.2 gm	545 mg

SALAD
DRESSINGS

CREAMY LIGHT CAESAR DRESSING

Makes: 8 servings

The best-tasting low-fat Caesar salad dressing on the market still has 7 grams of fat per serving. This recipe has all the rich and tangy flavor that you crave, but at a fraction of the fat! A favorite in the diet study.

⅔ cup light sour cream
5 drained anchovy fillets (oil patted off with towel)
2 tablespoons fresh lemon juice
1–2 cloves garlic, pressed
1 teaspoon Worcestershire sauce
½ teaspoon black pepper, crushed
1 tablespoon minced shallot

1. Put all ingredients in blender.
2. Blend until smooth.

Kept refrigerated, this will last a week.

Serving size: 2 tablespoons

CAL	FAT	PROT	CARB	SODIUM
32	1.6 gm	1.5 gm	2.2 gm	113 mg

SPICY CITRUS DRESSING

Makes: 16 servings

This dressing has a tangy and slightly sweet flavor that works equally well with a chicken or melon salad. A complementary balance of flavors is achieved by using two different citrus juices—orange for sweetness and lime for acid. However, the secret ingredient that makes this dressing great is the lime zest. The peel contains a small amount of oil, which acts to both enhance and prolong the dressing's flavor when stored in the refrigerator.

2 teaspoons grated lime peel, green part only
½ cup freshly squeezed orange juice
2 green onions, tops only, minced (about 2 tablespoons)
juice of 1 fresh lime (about 3 tablespoons)
1 tablespoon minced cilantro
1 fresh serrano chili, seeded and minced
1 teaspoon sugar
1 tablespoon Dijon mustard
2 cloves garlic, minced
1 teaspoon ground cumin (for poultry salad)

1. Place all ingredients in a blender.
2. Blend until smooth.
3. Refrigerate for 3 hours to let the flavors "marry."

Kept refrigerated, this will last 4 to 5 days.

Serving size: 2 tablespoons

CAL	FAT	PROT	CARB	SODIUM
16	0.4 gm	0.7 gm	2.5 mg	62 mg

CREAMY TARRAGON DRESSING

Makes: 11 servings

This dressing has such a rich and creamy texture, you would never guess it's low-fat. The balsamic vinegar lends a mellow sweetness and the herbs provide a garden-fresh flavor that enhances the taste of salads, vegetables and fish!

1 clove garlic, minced
pinch of kosher salt
1 cup low-fat sour cream
3 tablespoons balsamic vinegar
2 teaspoons fresh lemon juice
1 teaspoon Dijon mustard
2 teaspoons sugar
1½ tablespoons fresh minced tarragon (can substitute 2 teaspoons
*   dried tarragon)*
½ tablespoon minced chives
½ teaspoon fresh cracked pepper

1. Put garlic and salt in a mortar. Grind to a smooth paste.
2. Place all ingredients in a blender and puree until smooth.
3. Place in refrigerator for 3 hours to let the flavors "marry."

*Kept refrigerated, this will last 4 to 5 days.

Serving size: 2 tablespoons

CAL	FAT	PROT	CARB	FIBER	SODIUM
33	1.5 gm	0.8 gm	3.4 gm	0.1 gm	54 mg

TIP: If you're in a hurry, just place all the ingredients in the blender and blend until smooth.

CREAMY DILL DRESSING

Makes: 10 servings

This dressing has a creamy texture and slightly sweet flavor. The fat content has been reduced by combining nonfat and low-fat sour cream, so you can be more liberal with your portion. The dill complements the flavor of salads, and this dressing is also wonderful used as a sauce over boiled potatoes or salmon.

½ cup low-fat sour cream
½ cup nonfat sour cream
3 tablespoons balsamic vinegar
2 tablespoons fresh dill, chopped
1 tablespoon fresh chives, minced
1 teaspoon Dijon mustard
2 teaspoons sugar
1 clove garlic, chopped
1 teaspoon fresh cracked pepper
pinch of kosher salt

1. Combine all ingredients in a blender.
2. Blend until smooth.
3. Place in refrigerator for 3 hours to let the flavors "marry."

*Kept refrigerated, this will last 4 to 5 days.

Serving size: 2 tablespoons

CAL	FAT	PROT	CARB	FIBER	SODIUM
28	0.8 gm	1.7 gm	3.2 gm	0.1 gm	57 mg

Spicy Green Chili Salad Dressing

Makes: 13 servings

This chili-spiked salad dressing tastes anything but bland. It has a flavor that is reminiscent of the Green Goddess dressing but at a fraction of the fat! This recipe not only enhances the taste of a green salad, but makes a great topping for potatoes.

¼ cup light sour cream
¼ cup nonfat yogurt
1 tablespoon low-fat mayonnaise
4 fresh California green chilies, roasted, peeled and chopped (remove seeds and veins from 2 chilies to reduce "heat")
1 large green onion, chopped (green part only)
¼ teaspoon kosher salt
1 tablespoon fresh lemon juice
1 heaping teaspoon roasted garlic
1 teaspoon distilled white vinegar
dash of freshly cracked pepper
1 tablespoon fresh lemon juice

1. Add all ingredients in a blender.
2. Puree until smooth.
3. Chill for 3 hours to let the flavors "marry."
4. Add 1 tablespoon fresh lemon juice before serving.

Kept refrigerated, this will last a week.

Serving size: 2 tablespoons

CAL	FAT	PROT	CARB	FIBER	SODIUM
30	0.4 gm	0.8 gm	2.6 gm	2 gm	66 mg

SESAME GINGER SALAD DRESSING

Makes: 5 servings

If you've ever wondered how Chinese restaurants make their ginger salad dressing, the "secret ingredient" is preserved red ginger in syrup. This recipe has the authentic flavor of that signature dish, but is low-fat by reducing the traditional amounts of sesame seed oil. Since preserved red ginger is difficult to find, I substitute 1 teaspoon pureed white ginger (sold in small jars in well-stocked supermarkets).

> ¼ cup seasoned rice wine vinegar
> 1 teaspoon pureed white ginger
> ½ teaspoon light sesame oil
> 5 drops dark sesame chili oil
> 1 teaspoon white sugar
> 1 teaspoon sodium-reduced soy sauce

1. Put all ingredients in a blender and puree until smooth.
2. Put in refrigerator for several hours to let the flavors "marry."

*Kept refrigerated, this will last a week.

Serving size: 1 tablespoon

CAL	FAT	PROT	CARB	SODIUM
25	0.5 gm	0.1 gm	5.0 gm	217 mg

Blue Cheese Dressing

Makes: 17 servings

I love a good blue cheese dressing. Unfortunately, most full-fat products pack up to 16 grams of fat per serving! Nancy's Healthy Kitchen Lite Blue Cheese Dressing is the best commercial product of its kind on the market—it has that tangy flavor that I crave with a fraction of the fat. (It also lacks the funky after-taste that most other brands have.)

I found that when I added just a few fresh ingredients, this product rivaled any full-fat blue cheese dressing. The cottage cheese thickens its texture, while fresh lemon juice brightens the taste. Be sure to add plenty of fresh ground black pepper.

2 tablespoons Friendship Spreadable (1% Milkfat) Whipped Cottage
*   Cheese*
1 tablespoon fresh lemon juice
¼ teaspoon Worcestershire sauce
fresh cracked black pepper to taste
1 (16-oz.) container Nancy's Healthy Kitchen Lite Blue Cheese Dressing

1. Add cottage cheese, lemon juice, Worcestershire sauce and black pepper to contents of blue cheese dressing container. Stir. Allow product to sit for 24 hours so flavors can "marry."

Serving size: 2 tablespoons

CAL	FAT	PROT	CARB	SODIUM
28	1.4 gm	1.9 gm	1.9 gm	217 mg

TIP: Use Friendship's Whipped Cottage Cheese—it lacks the slimy texture and strange aftertaste that other 1% milk-fat cottage cheese products often have. The cottage cheese will also absorb the flavor of the blue cheese (like tofu), and give you more of that tangy blue cheese taste.

POULTRY DISHES

CARIBBEAN JERK CHICKEN

Makes: 4 servings

This recipe was cherished in the diet study. A client served this dish at a party, and everyone asked for the recipe. The "secret" to the success of this dish is using dark rum (molasses gives it a rich flavor) and fresh lime juice. Use leftovers in a chicken salad or sandwich the following day for a quick and easy lunch.

4 small chicken breasts w/bone, skin left on
2 oz. Meyer's Dark Rum (don't substitute light rum)
juice of 6 fresh limes
1 jar (12 oz.) Uncle Bum's Hot Jamaican Marinade

1. Pierce each breast with a fork 5 to 6 times (through the skin and into the meat).
2. In a small bowl, add rum and lime juice to marinade. Mix to blend.
3. Pour marinade over chicken and marinate for 2 hours (up to 6 hours).
4. Barbecue at 350° (skin side up) until juices run clear and meat is no longer pink—about 30 minutes. Remove the skin before eating.

Serving size: 1 chicken breast (4 ounces cooked meat)

CAL	FAT	PROT	FIBER	SODIUM
142	3.1 gm	26.7 gm	0.0 gm	64 mg

CHINESE CHICKEN SALAD

Makes: 1 serving

A typical restaurant Chinese chicken salad comes in at 1,100 calories. This reduced-calorie rendition substitues "oven-fried" wonton skins for the crispy noodles to provide crunch, while the sesame ginger dressing uses just the right balance of ginger, healthy oils and sugar to pack a flavorful punch. Look for the puréed ginger in the produce or ethnic section of your supermarket—it comes in a jar. A great dish for using up leftover roasted or grilled chicken!

3 wonton skins
Tryson House All Natural Oriental Mist Flavor Spray
1½ cups heart of romaine lettuce, sliced ¼-inch thick (about ½ head)
3 ounces leftover shredded Caribbean Jerk Chicken (or skinless cooked
* chicken breast)*
⅓ cup sliced red bell pepper
⅓ cup shredded carrots
⅓ cup green onions (tops only), thinly sliced (about ½ bunch)
¼ cup chopped cilantro (about ½ small bunch)
2–3 red jalapenos, chopped
3 tablespoons Sesame Ginger Salad Dressing

1. Prepare Sesame Ginger Salad Dressing (to follow).

2. Preheat toaster oven to 350°.

3. Stack three wonton skins on top of each other, and slice into ¼-inch lengths.

4. Line a baking pan with foil. Separate and lay wonton skins on foil-lined pan. Spray wonton skins with Tryson House All Natural Oriental Mist Flavor Spray (or canola oil nonstick spray) for 2 seconds.

5. Place wonton skins in oven and bake till crisp. Remove from oven and cool.

6. Put lettuce, chicken, bell pepper, carrots, green onions, cilantro and chilies in a bowl and toss with Sesame Ginger Salad Dressing.

7. Top with "oven-fried" wonton skins.

*These numbers denote a serving of salad with dressing.

CAL	FAT	PROT	CARB	FIBER	SODIUM
357	6.9 gm	30.2 gm	40.9 gm	5.2 gm	837 mg

Sesame Ginger Salad Dressing

Makes: 6 tablespoons

¼ cup seasoned rice wine vinegar
1 teaspoon pureed ginger
½ teaspoon light sesame oil
5 drops dark sesame oil
1 teaspoon white sugar
1 teaspoon sodium-reduced soy sauce

1. Put all ingredients in a blender and puree until smooth.

MEXICAN HERBED POACHED CHICKEN BREAST

Makes: 6 servings

It's hard to imagine that cooking a chicken breast in liquid can create dry, tough meat but it often does. The secret to savory, succulent breast meat is using a gentle heat for a brief period of time, then allowing the breast meat to "finish" cooking in its own broth ensures the meat remains tender, flavorful and moist. Use poached chicken breast in soft tacos, stuffed in a pita or add to a salad for a quick and easy lunch.

> 6 cups water
> 1 medium white onion, peeled and quartered
> ½ teaspoon thyme
> 1 teaspoon Mexican oregano
> 1 large carrot, halved
> 5 black peppercorns
> 1 bay leaf
> 1 large skinless, chicken breast (about 1 pound)
> 2 cloves garlic, lightly crushed
> 1 guajillo chili

1. In a 2-quart saucepan, add water, onion, thyme, oregano, carrot, peppercorns, bay leaf, garlic and chili and bring to a boil.
2. Add chicken breast and allow broth to return to a boil.
3. Reduce heat to medium-low and simmer for 4 minutes.
4. Remove pot from heat.
5. Cover pot and allow chicken to cool in its own broth to room temperature.
6. Place chicken on a cutting board. Remove skin and meat from bone and shred with two forks. (You should have about 1½ cups of meat.)

Serving size: 3 ounces

CAL	FAT	PROT	CARB	FIBER	SODIUM
142	3 gm	26.4 gm	0 gm	0 gm	63 mg

TIP: Chicken develops a richer flavor when it's poached in stock, rather than water. Strain and freeze the stock to use in the next batch of poached chicken.

SOFT CHICKEN TACOS

Makes: 1 serving

Soft chicken tacos are ideally suited for a low-fat diet, and they make a quick lunch or light main course for dinner.

¼ cup finely chopped cilantro
½ cup shredded lettuce
2 6-inch corn tortillas
3 ounces of poached chicken (can substitute
  skinless, roasted chicken breast)
½ cup Salsa Cruda (see recipe under Salsas)

1. In a medium bowl, mix cilantro with shredded lettuce.
2. Preheat oven at 350°. Wrap tortillas in foil and heat for 15 minutes (tortillas should be soft and flexible).
3. Place chicken, lettuce mixture and Salsa Cruda in warm tortilla.
4. Fold tortilla in half and serve.

CAL	FAT	PROT	CARB	FIBER	SODIUM
341	5.9 gm	29.4 gm	36 gm	4.4 gm	359 mg

MEXICAN CHICKEN SALAD WITH AVOCADO SALSA

Makes: 1 serving

Full of complex flavors, this hearty salad is a meal in itself.

> *3 ounces Mexican Herbed Poached Chicken*
> *Breast (see recipe) (can substitute roasted,*
> *skinless chicken breast or Caribbean Jerk*
> *Chicken [see recipe])*
> *½ cup canned pinto beans, heated in bean*
> *broth and drained*
> *1½ cups sliced romaine lettuce, ¼ inch slice*
> *½ cup Salsa Cruda (see recipe)*
> *¼ cup Avocado Salsa (see recipe)*

1. Place sliced lettuce on a plate.

2. Top with beans, chicken and Salsa Cruda.

3. Pour Avocado Salsa over salad and serve.

CAL	FAT	PROT	CARB	FIBER	SODIUM
324	8.4 gm	34.4 gm	29.85 gm	11.45 gm	898 mg

SEAFOOD

BROILED SALMON WITH CHIPOTLE CREAM SAUCE

Makes: 1 serving

The chipotle cream sauce uses evaporated milk, chicken stock and a reduction technique to achieve the taste and texture of a full-fat cream. The chipotle chili imparts a sweet and smoky taste—the perfect counterpoint flavor to the rich taste of the salmon. A deliciously simple and satisfying dish.

4 oz. fillet Norwegian or Atlantic salmon, center cut
⅛ cup chicken stock, fat removed
1 clove garlic, pressed
pinch of kosher salt
½ cup low-fat evaporated milk
½ tablespoon chipotle adobo sauce (sauce that chilies are packed in)

1. Preheat broiler.
2. Cook fish until flesh is turning opaque and flakes easily with a fork (approximately 3 to 4 minutes).
3. Preheat an 8-inch nonstick pan on medium heat. Combine stock, garlic and a pinch of salt. Sauté until tender.
4. Add milk and chipotle sauce to nonstick pan. Increase heat to high, bring liquid to a boil and shake the pan back and forth as the liquid bubbles until liquid is reduced by half. About ¼ cup of thick, viscous sauce should remain in pan.
5. Add another pinch of salt if needed. Shake pan back and forth two times.
6. Remove sauce from heat and pour over fish.

CAL	FAT	PROT	CARB	FIBER	SODIUM
270	9.3 gm	30.8 gm	13.8 gm	0.1 gm	608 mg

GRILLED SWORDFISH WITH ROASTED PEPPER SAUCE

Makes: 1 serving

The smoky, sweet flavor of the roasted red pepper sauce complements the meaty texture of the grilled swordfish. The mace and cloves add a sweet flavor and the guajillo chili lends a spicy, citrus tone, making this a wonderful dish for summer entertaining.

> 5 oz. swordfish fillet
> 1 teaspoon olive oil
> ¼ teaspoon cumin
> ¼ teaspoon mace
> 1 guajillo chili, rehydrated and pulp removed
> 1 teaspoon ancho chili powder
> ¼ teaspoon cloves
> ½ cup chicken stock, fat removed
> 1 garlic, minced
> 1 tablespoon minced onion
> 1 cup red bell pepper, roasted, peeled, seeded and chopped
>   (approximately 2 peppers)
> 1 teaspoon minced cilantro
> pinch of kosher salt

*To roast the peppers, place over a gas flame and turn as the skin blisters and chars. Wrap pepper in a moist cloth towel until it cools. Peel skin off with your fingers; do not rinse with water as this will remove some of the flavor.

1. Preheat broiler. Broil fish until just opaque and browned on top (about 7 minutes per inch of thickness).

2. Preheat 10-inch nonstick pan on medium-low heat. Add oil and shake skillet to distribute oil. Add spices and chili. Sauté until fragrant.

3. Add stock, garlic, onion and roasted peppers. Increase heat to high until mixture boils. Reduce liquid by half.

4. Transfer vegetable mixture to a blender and puree.

5. Return vegetable mixture to pan and heat on medium heat until hot.

6. Add minced cilantro and salt. Shake pan back and forth several times to blend.

7. Pour over fish and serve.

CAL	FAT	PROT	CARB	FIBER	SODIUM
297	11.5 gm	32.1 gm	17.5 gm	4.7 gm	543 mg

CHILEAN SEA BASS WITH TEQUILA LIME SAUCE

Makes: 1 serving

This is an easy and wonderfully balanced recipe. The tequila, garlic and shallots impart sweetness and depth, and the fresh lime juice imparts a refreshing accent.

> 4 oz. Chilean sea bass fillet, tail end
> juice of 1 fresh lemon
> ¼ cup tequila
> 5–6 cloves garlic, chopped
> 1 tablespoon minced shallot
> juice of ½ fresh lime
> pinch of kosher salt
> 1 tablespoon minced cilantro

1. Preheat oven to broil.
2. Rinse fish with lemon juice to clean and pat dry.
3. Place fish in broiler pan. Broil until fish is lightly browned on top and is just turning white (about 4–6 minutes).
4. While fish is broiling, preheat an 8-inch nonstick skillet on medium heat. Add tequila, garlic and shallots. Sauté until tender. Reduce the amount of liquid by shaking the pan back and forth to create a thick sauce—about 5 tablespoons.
5. Add lime juice, kosher salt and shake the pan back and forth (four times).
6. Add cilantro at the end of this reduction process to keep its color and flavor fresh.
7. Pour sauce over the fish and serve.

CAL	FAT	PROT	CARB	FIBER	SODIUM
173	3 g	28.1 gm	7.5 gm	0.5 gm	397 mg

CURRY CRUSTED TROUT

Makes: 1 serving

1 small trout fillet (about 5 ounces)
juice of ½ fresh lemon
1 tablespoon Paul Prudhomme's Seafood Magic Seasoning Blend
olive oil nonstick spray
1 teaspoon Madras curry powder
⅛ teaspoon ground ginger

1. Rinse fish with lemon juice and pat dry.
2. Mix seasoning blend, curry powder and ginger.
3. Season both sides of fish with seasoning blend.
4. Heat medium nonstick pan on medium-high heat until hot.
5. Spray (one second) with olive oil nonstick spray.
6. Add fish and cook until a crust forms (about one minute).
7. Flip fish over and cook until done.

CAL	FAT	PROT	CARB	FIBER	SODIUM
128	9.8 gm	29.9 gm	2.6 gm	.7 gm	179 mg

SEARED SHRIMP WITH ANCHO CHILIES

Makes: 2 servings

This dish is an extravaganza for the eye as well as the palate. The concentrated ancho chili vinegar (resembles a robust balsamic) imparts a ruby hue to the shrimp while enhancing their delicate, sweet taste. The arbol chili is added to lend a touch of heat. It's important to turn the shrimp once the sugars in the vinegar caramelize. Otherwise, this dish takes on the bitter taste of burnt sugar.

> 1 cup water
> 2 cups Japanese seasoned rice wine vinegar
> 2 ancho chilies, stemmed, seeded and cut into ¼-inch strips
> 10 shrimp (3.5 ounces per serving)
> 1 teaspoon lemon juice
> 2 cloves garlic, minced
> 2 arbol chilies
> 1 teaspoon garlic-and-àrbol-flavored olive oil
> pinch of kosher salt
> Ancho chili vinegar

1. Put water, Japanese seasoned rice wine vinegar and ancho chilies in a pot and bring to a boil.

2. Reduce to a simmer. Press chilies against the side of pot with the back side of a spoon several times to release color and flavor. Reduce mixture until the color of the vinegar matches a balsamic vinegar (takes approximately 15 minutes and makes 2 cups). Strain and set aside.

Shrimp

1. Heat a 10-inch nonstick pan on medium heat and spray (one time) with an olive nonstick spray.

2. Add 1 teaspoon of olive oil and shake pan to coat. Add garlic-àrbol chilies and pinch of kosher salt and sauté for 30 seconds and then add shrimp.

3. When shrimp turn pink, flip them over and add ⅛-cup ancho chili vinegar. Stir to coat.

4. Let vinegar reduce until it caramelizes; shrimp should be ruby-colored flecked with black.

Serving size: 7.35 ounces

CAL	FAT	PROT	CARB	FIBER	SODIUM
158	2.4 gm	21.9 gm	12.2 gm	1.6 gm	612 mg

CURRIED TUNA SANDWICH

Makes: 1 serving

A restaurant tuna fish sandwich can pack 700 calories and 50 grams of fat! Loaded with full-fat mayo, what *should* be a healthy sandwich is transported into the nutritional realm of a double bacon cheeseburger! Substituting nonfat mayo isn't an option either—its "off" taste and texture is a compromise most people aren't willing to make. However, if you use this product as a base and add bold spices and fruit—it works! In this recipe, the curry picks up the flavor while the grapes thicken its texture. The one caveat with using nonfat mayo as a binding agent—eat the food right after you prepare it since the mayonnaise breaks down quickly and gets "watery."

In a simple dish like tuna salad, technique makes a huge difference. First and foremost, use the best-tasting tuna on the market, Starkist's Solid White Albacore Tuna. Drain the tuna in a mesh colander, then crumble it between your fingers until you get a fine, even texture. This additional step ensures that you get a smooth-textured salad. Finally, season the drained tuna with kosher salt and fresh cracked black pepper before you add the mayo, which brightens the flavor of the fish.

> ¼ cup nonfat mayo
> ¼ cup green seedless grapes
> ¼ teaspoon curry powder
> 1 can (3 oz.) Starkist's solid white albacore, water-packed
> kosher salt and pepper to taste
> ¼ cup chopped celery
> 2 slices whole wheat bread
> 4 slices tomato
> 4–5 thin slices hothouse cucumber
> 2 pickled jalapeno chilies, minced

1. Put nonfat mayo and grapes in a blender, and blend until smooth.

2. Fold curry powder into mayo mixture with a fork until incorporated.

3. Open can of tuna, and drain in a mesh colander. Break down the larger chunks of tuna with your fingers until a fine and even texture is achieved.

4. Season the tuna with a dash of salt and fresh cracked pepper.

5. Transfer drained, seasoned tuna to a bowl and add chopped celery until evenly blended.

6. Fold curried mayo into the tuna.

7. Place tuna on whole wheat bread and top with tomato, cucumber and minced, pickled peppers.

CAL	FAT	PROT	CARB	FIBER	SODIUM
291	4.2 gm	25.3 gm	42.9 gm	4.8 gm	1,021 mg

HOT HINTS: Nonfat mayo breaks down rapidly and makes the tuna salad "watery." You'll get the best results if you eat the sandwich right after you prepare it—do not store the finished tuna salad in the fridge.

CURRIED TUNA SALAD

Makes: 1 serving

In this recipe, a small amount of light sour cream is added to the nonfat mayo to enhance both its taste and texture. You'll get the best results if you eat the sandwich right after you prepare it, since nonfat mayo breaks down rapidly and makes the tuna salad "watery."

⅛ cup light sour cream
¼ cup nonfat mayonnaise
1 teaspoon curry powder
1 can (3 oz.) of Starkist's Solid White Albacore Tuna, water-packed
kosher salt and pepper to taste
1 tablespoon minced shallot
1 medium apple, cored and chopped
1 tablespoon raisins
1½ cups sliced romaine lettuce
1–2 pickled jalapeno chilies, minced

1. In a small bowl, add nonfat mayo and light sour cream and blend until smooth.
2. Fold curry powder into mayo mixture with a fork until incorporated.
3. Open can of tuna, and drain in a mesh colander. Break down the larger chunks of tuna with your fingers until a fine and even texture is achieved.
4. Season the tuna with a dash of salt and fresh cracked pepper.
5. In a medium bowl, add tuna, shallots, apple and raisins. Toss until blended.
6. Fold curried mayo into the tuna.
7. Place tuna on lettuce and top with minced, pickled peppers.

CAL	FAT	PROT	CARB	FIBER	SODIUM
333	6.2 gm	24.4 gm	48.2 gm	7.2+ gm	1,132 mg

BAGELS WITH SMOKED SALMON, CAPER CREAM CHEESE SPREAD AND TOMATOES

Makes: 1 serving

With a few changes, bagels, cream cheese and lox is transformed into a hearty and healthy meal. In this rendition, the healthy oils found in the smoked fish supply the fat, while the artery-clogging fat in the cream cheese has been slashed. Be sure to use a light squeeze of fresh lemon on the smoked salmon— acidity not only heightens the rather one-dimensional flavor of smoked food (salt and smoke) but also masks the saltiness of the fish.

1 2½–3-ounce plain bagel
2 tablespoons Caper Cream Cheese Spread (see recipe) (or plain
nonfat cream cheese)
1 oz. smoked salmon (preferably Norwegian, Scottish or Irish)
4 thin slices tomato
fresh lemon juice
1–2 pickled jalapenos, seeded and minced
2 thin slices red onion (optional)

1. Split and lightly toast bagel.

2. Spread Caper Cream Cheese Spread on bagel.

3. Place one slice (½ oz.) of salmon on each bagel half.

4. Squeeze a small amount of fresh lemon over the smoked fish.

5. Top with tomato, red onion and pickled jalapenos.

CAL	FAT	PROT	CARB	FIBER	SODIUM
286	3.7 gm	18.5 gm	44.3 gm	3 gm	871 mg

SIDES
AND SALADS

DRY ROASTED CURRIED POTATOES

Makes: 3 servings

Leaving the skin on the potatoes during cooking not only preserves nutrients but flavor. There are two secrets to this technique. One is to use a gentle boil and keep the potatoes barely covered with water during the cooking process. (If you use a rapid boil or use too much water, the potato skins will split.) Two, keep an eye on the potatoes during cooking—you may need to add a bit of water to keep them covered. A good way to test if the potatoes are done is to insert a bamboo grilling stick into the potato—a perfectly cooked potato will be soft in the center. Although this technique will take longer than the conventional boiling method—it's worth it! However, if you're short on time—just peel and boil the spuds.

Butter-flavored nonstick spray
2 medium russet baking potatoes (organic potatoes have the best flavor)
1 tablespoon Madras curry powder
2 tablespoons Chef Paul Prudhomme's Seafood Magic Seasoning Blend
fresh ground pepper to taste
1 teaspoon fresh minced ginger
2 seranno chilies, minced
1 tablespoon minced cilantro

1. In a 6-quart pot, add potatoes and enough water to just cover potatoes.

2. Heat on high heat to a rapid boil.

3. Reduce heat to a gentle boil, and cook potatoes until done—about 45 minutes.

4. Remove potatoes from water and cool.

5. Peel and dice potatoes (½-inch dice; about 2 cups)

6. Heat 8-inch heavy nonstick pan on medium-high heat for one minute until hot.

7. Spray (one second) with butter-flavored nonstick spray.

8. Add diced potatoes. Sprinkle with curry powder, Seafood Magic Seasoning Blend, black pepper and ginger.

9. Spray (½ second) top of potatoes with butter-flavored spray. Let a crust form, and gently shake pan.

10. Add minced serrano chilies. Shake and gently flip potatoes till a second crust forms (let potatoes sit a bit between shakes to ensure a crust forms).

11. Top with minced cilantro.

Serving size: ½ cup

CAL	FAT	PROT	CARB	FIBER	SODIUM
114	0.7 gm	2.7 gm	26 gm	3 gm	106 mg

FRESH CORN WITH LIME AND CHILIES

Makes: 4 servings

In Mexico, corn on the cob is seasoned with fresh lime juice and chili powder, instead of melted butter. Although I had my doubts about this dish, I was hooked after the first bite—this magical flavor combination enhanced the sweet flavor of the corn much better than butter! A wonderful chili seasoning for corn is Chef Moritos's Pikos Pikosos Chili Powder, which can be obtained in Latin markets or ordered online: E-mail: *INFO@monterreyfoodproducts.com* or *www.monterreyfoodproducts.com*. However, you can also make your own seasoning blend.

The secret to perfectly cooked corn is not to boil it—a high heat toughens the proteins. You'll get much better results if you use a gentle heat instead. First, bring the water to a boil, then add your fresh, shucked corn. When the water returns to a boil, immediately turn off the heat and cover the pot for 15 minutes. If the corn is more than two days old, add ¼ cup of white sugar to the cooking water. The sugar not only tenderizes the corn, but sweetens it.

½ teaspoon àrbol chili powder
½ teaspoon kosher salt
2 large fresh ears of corn (can use 4 small ears of corn)
2 fresh limes

1. Grind àrbol chili powder and salt in a coffee grinder. Set aside.

2. Bring a large pot of water to a boil and add corn.

3. When water returns to a boil, immediately turn off heat and cover pot with lid for 15 minutes.

4. Remove corn from pot. Squeeze fresh lime juice over corn and season with chili powder.

Serving size: ½ large ear of corn; 1 small ear of corn

CAL	FAT	PROT	CARB	FIBER	SODIUM
45	0.5 gm	1.4 gm	10.5 gm	1.2 gm	303 mg

CHARRO BEANS

Makes: 7 servings

This dish is called "cowboy beans" in Mexico. It is broth-based, which makes it much lower in fat compared to refried beans. Morita chilies are added to impart a hot smoky flavor—you'll swear someone slipped a ham hock into the pot! This simple recipe is wonderful when you don't have time to cook.

4 cups pinto beans (2 15-ounce cans)
4 morita chilies, whole (can substitute 2 chipotle chilies)
1 cup water
¼ cup chopped white onion, soaked in ice water for 10 minutes (reduces the onion's "bite")
¼ cup minced cilantro

1. Put beans, chilies and water in a 2-quart pot.
2. Heat on medium heat until liquid reduces by half (approximately 15 minutes).
3. Remove morita chilies.
4. Drain onions.
5. Place beans in a bowl and top with onion and cilantro.

Serving size: ⅓ cup

CAL	FAT	PROT	CARB	FIBER	SODIUM
48.5	0.2 gm	2.85 gm	9.15 gm	3.4 gm	254 mg

TOASTED MEXICAN-STYLE RICE

Makes: 7 servings

This a low-fat version of the classic Mexican-style rice. The fat is reduced by toasting (instead of frying) the rice before adding the stock. Caramelizing the starches adds depth and gives the rice a wonderfully nutty flavor and fluffy texture.

1 cup long-grain white rice
2 cups heated chicken stock, fat removed
½ medium white onion, chopped to ¼-inch dice
1–2 cloves garlic, chopped fine
1 small tomato, seeded and chopped to ¼-inch dice
½–1 teaspoon kosher salt
2 tablespoons minced cilantro

1. Put rice in a baking pan and toast in oven at 350° until golden brown. Shake pan back and forth several times to ensure even heating. (An alternative method is to put rice in a heavy 10-inch nonstick skillet and cook at a medium heat, shaking or stirring the rice several times until golden brown.)

2. Pour hot stock in a 2-quart pot.

3. Add onion, toasted rice, garlic, tomato and salt.

4. Bring mixture to a boil.

5. Cover pot and reduce heat to low. Cook for 20–22 minutes.

6. Add cilantro and toss.

* For herbed rice, omit the tomato and cilantro. Use dried tarragon instead, and add at step #2.

Serving size: ½ cup

CAL	FAT	PROT	CARB	FIBER	SODIUM
108	0.3 gm	2.5 gm	23.3 gm	1.1+ gm	451 mg

BROCCOLI SLAW

Makes: 4 servings

Broccoli belongs to a group of vegetables called the cruciferous family. It contains phytochemicals, indoles and sulforaphanes, which provide protection against cancer. The good news is a high concentration of these chemicals is also found in the stems, which have a sweeter taste and lack the bitter bite that many people find offensive in the florets. The secret to the success of this dish is using a small julienne cut, and then marinating the stems in rice wine vinegar, which softens their woody texture. Works well as a vegetable side dish or on a turkey sandwich instead of lettuce.

> 6 broccoli stems, washed, peeled and sliced ⅛-inch thick (use a hand
>   slicing machine)
> ½ cup seasoned rice wine vinegar
> 2 serrano chilies, minced
> ½ red bell pepper, diced
> ½ yellow bell pepper, diced
> 1 teaspoon sugar

1. Put broccoli stems in a bowl and cover with rice wine vinegar till the stems soften (about 20 minutes).

2. Add peppers and sugar. Marinate for an additional 10 minutes to let the flavors "marry."

Kept refrigerated, this will last 1 to 2 days.

Serving size: ½ cup

CAL	FAT	PROT	CARB	FIBER	SODIUM
33	0.4 gm	2.9 gm	6.7 gm	3 gm	24 mg

TABOOLEH

Makes: 7 servings

This is a variation of the classic Middle Eastern dish, tabooleh. The base of this salad is cracked wheat, which makes it a filling dish.

> ¾ cup boiling water
> 1½ cups medium bulgar (#2)
> 1 shallot, minced
> juice of 2 lemons
> 1 cup minced parsley
> 1 roma tomato, chopped
> 1 teaspoon kosher salt
> 1 tablespoon extra virgin olive oil
> 1 clove garlic, minced
> ¼ cup chopped picking (kerbie or Persian) cucumber
> 1 cup garbanzo beans, marinated in ½ cup freshly
>   squeezed lemon juice for 24 hours

1. Mix water and bulgar.
2. Cover until cool.
3. Fold in next 9 ingredients.
4. Add beans and mix.
5. Chill for 5 hours.

*Kept refrigerated, this will last 4 days.

Serving size: ½ cup

CAL	FAT	PROT	CARB	FIBER	SODIUM
171	2.8 gm	5.8 gm	33.2 gm	8.1+ gm	449 mg

RICE VERDE

Makes: 9 servings

This a low-fat version of the classic Mexican rice dish, arroz verde. The fat is reduced by toasting (instead of frying) the rice before adding the stock. The roasted poblano chili is added to impart a delightful color and smoky flavor.

> 1 cup long-grain white rice
> 2 cups heated chicken stock, fat removed
> ½ medium white onion, chopped
> 1 clove garlic, minced
> 4 poblano chilies, roasted, peeled and chopped
> 1 teaspoon kosher salt
> ½ small bunch cilantro (leaves only), chopped

1. Put rice in a baking pan and toast in a 350°F oven, shaking the pan back and forth several times until golden brown. (An alternative method is to put rice in a heavy dry pan, and cook at a medium heat while stirring until golden brown.)
2. Put hot stock in a 2-quart pot.
3. Add onion, rice, garlic, chilies and salt.
4. Bring to a boil.
5. Cover pot and reduce heat to low. Cook for 20 to 22 minutes.
6. Remove from heat. Add cilantro.
7. Mix with fork and serve.

Serving size: ½ cup

CAL	FAT	PROT	CARB	FIBER	SODIUM
91	0.2 gm	2.2 gm	19.7 gm	1.1+ gm	482 mg

TROPICAL FRUIT SALAD

Makes: 16 servings

Many people don't eat enough fruit—they grab sugary pastries and ice cream to satisfy their "sweet tooth." This recipe uses lime juice, which increases the tongue's perception of sweetness, to enhance the flavor of fruit.

> 1 pineapple, peeled, cored and cut into ½-inch chunks
> 2 papayas, peeled, seeded and cut into ½-inch chunks
> juice of 4 fresh limes
> dash of cayenne chili powder (¼ teaspoon)
> 1 banana, peeled and cut into ½-inch slices
> 1 apple, cored and cut into ½-inch chunks
> 1 package strawberries, washed and cut in half
> 2 walnuts, chopped (optional)

1. Put pineapple and papaya in a bowl.

2. Squeeze lime juice over pineapple and papaya and marinate for 15 minutes. Sprinkle chili powder over fruit.

3. Mix bananas, apples, strawberries and walnuts. Toss gently.

4. Arrange pineapple and papaya around the edge of a large platter. Mound banana, apple and strawberry mixture in center.

5. Chill and serve.

Serving size: ½ cup

CAL	FAT	PROT	CARB	FIBER	SODIUM
48	0.4 gm	0.6 gm	11.9 gm	1.8 gm	2 mg

Although putting an acid over fruit may sound strange, participants in the diet study were surprised how this "trick" made eating fruit a more enjoyable experience! This technique works in a similar fashion to salting watermelon.

REFRIED BLACK BEANS

Makes: 2 servings

Traditionally, refried beans derive their rich flavor and creamy texture from lard. This recipe uses a reduction technique to concentrate flavors, and replaces that artery-clogging saturated fat with roasted salsa, ground chili and cumin to create a truly soul-satisfying side dish.

2 medium plum tomatoes, seeded and chopped
¼ small white onion, minced
2 medium cloves garlic, pressed or minced
pinch of kosher salt
½ can black beans and their liquid
¼ teaspoon ground cumin
1 teaspoon ground New Mexican chili powder
2 teaspoons cotija cheese (can substitute Greek feta cheese)

Roasted salsa

1. Heat a heavy 8-inch nonstick pan on medium heat until hot.
2. Add tomatoes, onions and garlic. Dry roast, stirring occasionally, until slightly charred. Remove and set aside.
3. In a mortar, add several pinches of kosher salt and roasted tomato mixture. Grind to a chunky, thick paste.

Refried beans

1. Heat a heavy 8-inch nonstick pan on medium heat until hot.
2. Add beans, bean liquid, roasted salsa, cumin and ground chili.
3. Increase heat to medium-high. Fry the beans until a soft crust forms on the bottom of the pan. Mash the beans, bean liquid and salsa with a potato masher each time a crust forms until a thick, slightly chunky texture is achieved. The beans should be thick, but not dry.
4. Top with cheese.

Serving size: ½ cup

CAL	FAT	PROT	CARB	FIBER	SODIUM
95	2.1 gm	5.7 gm	20.2 gm	6.3 gm	528 mg

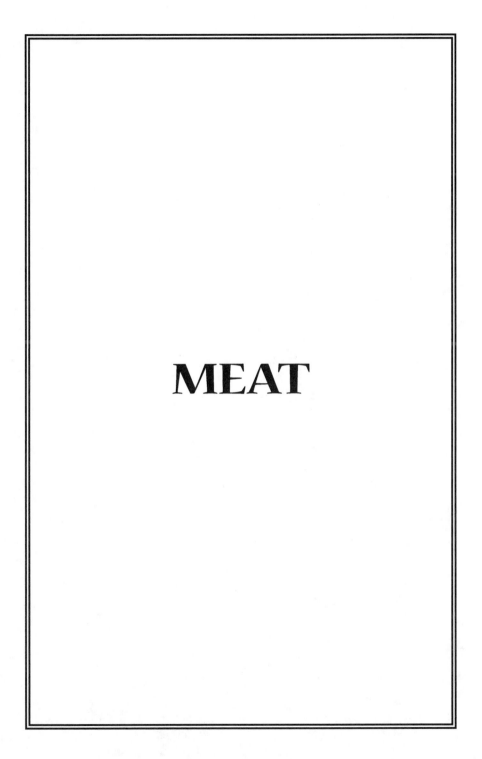

MEAT

BRAISED BRISKET WITH ONION GRAVY

Makes: 11 servings

This recipe uses a slow, moist heat to soften the tough texture of the meat. Although I've added other ingredients to try to improve it, it really tastes best with just three ingredients. Everyone who has tried this recipe just loves it, and you don't have to be a chef to prepare it. This recipe freezes well, and leftovers make a great soft-meat taco! Since this is a fatty meat, reserve it for holidays and special occasions.

> 1 package Lipton onion soup mix
> 3 pounds beef brisket (center cut), visible
>   fat removed
> 1 medium onion, thinly sliced
> water to cover

1. Preheat oven to 325°.
2. Place meat on top of a large piece (four times the size of the meat) of heavy-duty aluminum foil.
3. Sprinkle Lipton onion soup mix on top and around sides of meat. Place sliced onions around meat. Add enough water (about 4 cups) just to cover the meat.
4. Make a tent with the foil, crimping the edges so that the meat, onions, water and soup mix are completely enclosed. Place foil tent in a heavy roasting pan.
5. Place the foil tent containing meat, water, onions and soup mix in oven. Cook for 3½ to 4 hours.
6. Remove the foil packet from the oven and cool for 30 minutes to finish cooking.
7. Strain onions from gravy and pour the gravy into a fat separator (a container which separates the juice from the fat).
8. Slice the meat against the grain into ¼-inch slices and top with gravy.

* You should check the meat every 2 hours to see if it needs more water.

Serving size: 3 ounces of meat with 2 tablespoons of gravy

CAL	FAT	PROT	CARB	FIBER	SODIUM
192	8.7 gm	25.8 gm	0.6 gm	0.0 gm	183 mg

HAMBURGER

Makes: 1 serving

The typical 7-ounce restaurant burger packs close to 1,000 calories, 60 grams of fat and 900 milligrams of sodium. If you thought a juicy burger is verboten on a low-fat diet—think again! By using low-fat ingredients and specialized cooking techniques, this American culinary icon is transformed into a much healthier meal.

Start with a lean cut of meat (5 to 7 percent fat), and limit your portion size to 4 ounces. If your market does not carry this product, have your butcher trim and grind a sirloin steak. The secret to using this lean cut of meat is twofold: shape and temperature. Slightly indenting the center of the patty ensures that you wind up with a moist and evenly cooked burger. If the patty is uniformly flat, the meat juices pulled inward during the cooking process create a raw, bulging center and dry edges. Don't skip this step—it's crucial for good results. It's also important that you preheat your nonstick pan at a high heat for 60 seconds, which creates crust and seals in the flavorful meat juices (a medium-heat steams, rather that sears, the meat).

Other burger caveats include: not cooking the meat past the medium-rare stage and avoid flattening the patty with a spatula while cooking. Use a spatula only to flip the burger—after a crust has formed. While this healthy rendition allows you to indulge your burger craving, limit this dish to several times per month.

Tryson House Mesquite Nonstick
   Flavor Spray
1 tablespoon fat-free mayo
1 teaspoon ketchup
1 teaspoon pickle relish
4 oz. 5% fat hamburger

1 small, plain bun
1–2 slices tomato
shredded hearts of romaine lettuce
1 slice onion
1 teaspoon chipotle sauce (spicy
   tomato sauce chilies are packed in)

Secret Sauce

1. In a small bowl, mix nonfat mayo, ketchup, chipotle sauce (sauce in canned chipotle chilies) and relish.

Burger

1. Heat a heavy 8-inch nonstick pan on high heat for 1 minute.

2. Shape burger patty (3½ inches side and ½-inch high). Using your thumbs, slightly indent the burger in the center to create a circle (about 1 inch in diameter and ¼-inch deep).

3. Spray the nonstick pan (one-second spray) and meat (½-second spray) with Tryson House Mesquite Nonstick Flavor Spray. Cook until a crust forms—about 2 minutes.

4. Flip the patty and cook for an additional 1½ minutes. Remove patty and season with a pinch of kosher salt.

5. Spread 1 tablespoon of secret sauce on top half of bun.

6. Place meat patty on bottom bun and layer with tomatoes, shredded lettuce and onion slices.

CAL	FAT	PROT	CARB	FIBER	SODIUM
324	8.5 gm	30.1 gm	30.1 gm	2.0+ gm	591 mg

SOUPS

SMOKY CHIPOTLE CORN CHOWDER

Makes: 1 serving

This soup tastes rich but contains no saturated fat. The starch in the corn gives this soup a thick texture, and the chicken stock combined with the skim milk mimic the rich taste of cream. The wonderful smoky flavor imparted by the chipotle chilies is enhanced by adding a drop of liquid mesquite right before serving. This soup is comfort food on a cold day!

Tryson House Mesquite Nonstick Spray
¼ medium onion, chopped
½ cup chicken stock, fat removed or substitute ½ cup Imagine Natural
  Organic Free Range Chicken Broth
2 ears fresh yellow corn
2 tablespoons water
2 cups chicken stock, fat removed or substitute Imagine Natural
  Organic Free Range Chicken Broth
1 teaspoon liquid from chipotle adobe (chipotle chili in tomato sauce)
⅓ can evaporated skim milk
½ guajillo chili, soaked and the inside pulp scraped out (optional)
¼ teaspoon liquid mesquite flavoring (look in the spice section of the
  market)

1. Preheat an 8-inch nonstick skillet on medium-low heat. Spray skillet (twice) with Tryson House Mesquite Nonstick Spray. (Can substitute butter-flavored nonstick spray.)

2. Add onions and sauté until translucent. Add stock and reduce heat to low. Cook until onions are tender and stock has evaporated, about 15 minutes.

3. Microwave corn in a dish (covered with plastic wrap) in 2 tablespoons of water for 3 minutes and turn. Replace plastic wrap and continue to heat for approximately 8 minutes until tender. Remove corn from the cob.

4. Place corn in a blender with chicken stock, chipotle liquid, skim milk, onions and guajillo chili pulp. Blend until smooth.

5. Heat mixture in a 2-quart pot until hot.

6. Transfer to serving bowl. Add a drop of mesquite flavoring to hot soup, and stir to blend.

Serving size: Makes two 1-cup servings

CAL	FAT	PROT	CARB	FIBER	SODIUM
140.5	1.1 gm	7.45 gm	28.75 gm	2.65 gm	*783 mg

sodium content will be lower if homemade stock is used.

INDIAN ORANGE LENTIL SOUP WITH GINGER AND GARLIC

Makes: 12 servings

This exotic, savory soup is packed with health-promoting phytochemicals, fiber and flavor. Using a hand chopper and pureed ginger and garlic (packaged in a jar) cuts down on the prep time. For added convenience, freeze soup in single-serving containers and reheat in the microwave.

>	8 cups water
>	8 cups Swanson 99% Fat-Free Chicken Broth
>	1 pound dried red lentils
>	2 tablespoons pureed ginger root
>	2 tablespoons pureed garlic
>	1 medium onion, diced (1 heaping cup)
>	2 large carrots, diced (1 cup)
>	1¼ cups chopped celery (3 stalks)
>	3 large roma tomatoes, chopped (1 cup)
>	1 teaspoon turmeric powder
>	2 teaspoons curry powder
>	1 tablespoon red pepper flakes
>	1 teaspoon canola oil
>	2 medium green apples, peeled and shredded
>	1 teaspoon kosher salt
>	1 bunch cilantro, finely chopped

1. Bring water and stock to boil in large pot.
2. Add lentils and cook 5 minutes.
3. Add ginger, garlic, onion, carrots, celery, tomatoes, tumeric, curry, red pepper flakes, oil, apples and salt.

4. Bring to a boil, then reduce heat and simmer until soup is reduced by one fourth (about one hour).

5. Add cilantro and serve.

Kept refrigerated, this soup will last 3 to 4 days.

Serving size: 1 cup

CAL	FAT	PROT	CARB	FIBER	SODIUM
173	1.1 gm	12.2 gm	30.5 gm	6.1 gm	683 mg

WILD MUSHROOM AND BARLEY SOUP

Makes: 10 servings

Barley not only lowers cholesterol, but evens out insulin and blood sugar levels. Moreover, this wondergrain can help you lose weight! A recent study found levels of cholecystokinnin (a gut hormone that makes you feel full) were elevated for a longer period of time in people who ate a barley-based meal. Top this soup with ground arbol chilies for a soul-satisfying treat.

1 oz. dried porcini mushrooms
5 cups water
1 teaspoon Paul Prudhommes's Creole Vegetable Magic Seasoning
   (can substitute seafood blend)
1 tablespoon olive oil
1 teaspoon thyme
1½ cups chopped onion
1 large carrot, peeled and minced
2 stalks celery, ½-inch slice
1 8-oz. package button mushrooms, stems removed and quartered
2 fresh shiitake mushrooms, stems removed, ¼-inch slice
1 fresh oyster mushroom, ¼-inch slice
1 cup barley
2 15-oz. cans Swanson 99% Fat-Free Chicken Broth
1 cup 1% fat milk
toasted arbol or pequin chilies, ground to coarse flakes

1. Soak porcini mushrooms (covered) in 2 cups of boiling water for twenty minutes until rehydrated.

2. Heat a stockpot on medium heat. Add oil.

3. Add Creole seasoning blend, thyme, onions, carrots, celery and button, shiitake and oyster mushrooms. Stir and sauté until soft.

4. Add water, barley, stock and simmer for 1 hour.

5. Slowly add porcini mushrooms and 2 cups soaking from mushrooms. (Sand from the porcini mushrooms will collect at the bottom of the soaking bowl—leave the last few tablespoons of soaking liquid with sand in the bowl. Soaking liquid should be the color of coffee.)

6. Add milk.

7. Simmer for 20 minutes.

8. Grind chilies to a coarse powder in coffee grinder.

9. Put soup in bowl and top with ¼ to ½ teaspoon of chili.

Serving size: 1 cup

CAL	FAT	PROT	CARB	FIBER	SODIUM
329	1.9 gm	5.3 gm	20.8 gm	4.8+ gm	422 mg

CHEF JAMIE SHANNON'S ANCHO CHILI EGGPLANT SOUP

Makes: 6 servings

4 ancho chilies
3 qt. chicken stock (or substitute store-bought)
3 large eggplants
2 large onions
4 oz. peeled garlic (approx. 3 heads)
2 tablespoons olive oil
½ teaspoon curry powder
½ teaspoon white vinegar
salt and fresh cracked pepper to taste

1. Rehydrate chilies in chicken stock after they have been cleaned.

2. Peel eggplant and dice to approximately one inch. Peel onion and medium dice to one inch. Peel garlic, keeping toes whole. Toss with olive oil, salt and pepper.

3. Roast vegetables in oven at 350°F conventional oven and 300°F convection oven. Stir, do not burn; you want to caramelize vegetables and bring out the natural sugars, about 20 to 25 minutes. Do not take vegetables out of oven unless nicely brown.

4. While vegetables are roasting, place the stock on the stove in a large pot (at least a 2-gallon pot), with a heavy gauge bottom. Bring to a boil, then reduce to a simmer.

5. Add curry powder, roasted vegetables and simmer for ½ hour. Puree in blender. Add vinegar and stir.

6. Bring soup back to a simmer, adjust seasoning with salt and pepper.

7. If soup is not thick enough, reduce by simmering until consistency is right. If too thick, adjust with stock.

Note:
*The better the stock, the better the soup.
*Do not burn vegetables—brown them.
*You can always add more chilies.
*This soup tastes better if it's chilled overnight. It can double as a dip for pita bread.

Serving size: 1 cup

CAL	FAT	PROT	CARB	FIBER	SODIUM
75.5	2.5 gm	2.7 gm	11.45 gm	2.6+ gm	*570 mg

*The sodium content reflects commercially prepared chicken stock like Imagine Natural Organic Free Range Chicken Broth.

CARROT SOUP

Makes: 2 servings

This soup has a beautiful orange hue and a rich flavor. The orange juice enhances the sweet flavor of the carrots (the acid in the orange juice mellows as it is heated) and the guadillo chili imparts a spicy citrus tone. Don't forget to add the corn tortilla—it lends a subtle flavor and gives the soup a thick texture.

3 large carrots, peeled and chopped
2 cups chicken stock
½ teaspoon pureed ginger
1 large shallot, minced (about ⅙ cup)
½ corn tortilla, broken in small pieces
½ guadillo chili, soaked in hot water for 20 minutes, pulp removed
  (no seeds or veins)
¾ cup freshly squeezed orange juice
pinch of kosher salt

1. In a medium bowl, microwave carrots until tender (about 7–10 minutes).

2. Preheat an 8-inch nonstick pan on medium-low heat. Add ¼ cup of chicken stock, ginger and shallots and sauté until tender (about 8 minutes).

3. Put cooked carrots, corn tortilla, shallots/ginger mixture, chili and remaining stock in a blender. Blend until smooth.

4. Put vegetable mixture in a 2-quart pot. Add orange juice to carrot mixture and heat on medium heat until hot.

5. Add salt to taste.

CAL	FAT	PROT	CARB	FIBER	SODIUM
139	.5 gm	2.9 gm	29.5 gm	3.5 gm	196.5 mg

CHICKEN CONGEE

Makes: 1 serving

Ever wonder what to do with that leftover brown rice? Try this Asian-inspired soup, Chicken Congee. In Hong Kong, this hearty rice-based soup is cherished as a Dim Sum brunch item. And with a few changes, this soup is transformed into a much healthier meal by omitting the fried wontons, using brown rice and seasoning with Nampla (Thai fish-based soy sauce) rather than soy sauce. Nampla is a "secret" ingredient in many Thai dishes—it adds depth to a dish when used in small amounts. Moreover, this product is much lower in sodium than regular soy sauce. Look for it in the ethnic section of your supermarket.

> 1 cup pre-cooked brown rice (do not use basmati long-grain brown
>   rice—texture is too dry)
> 3 cups hot chicken stock (can substitute low-sodium canned
>   chicken stock)
> 2 oz. poached chicken breast (can substitute roasted chicken breast)
> ½ tablespoon Nampla
> 1 tablespoon thinly sliced green onion (green tops only), or
>   1 tablespoon minced chives

1. Put brown rice and stock in a blender and blend until you achieve an even consistency.

2. In a medium bowl, add rice mixture and poached chicken in a microwave. Heat on high for one minute and stir. Heat for an additional 1–2 minutes until hot.

3. Add Nampla and stir until incorporated into soup.

4. Top with green onions.

CAL	FAT	PROT	CARB	FIBER	SODIUM
380	3.8 gm	26.9 gm	51 gm	3.7 gm	140 mg

PASTA

PENNE WITH ROASTED EGGPLANT, TOMATO AND KALAMATA OLIVES

Makes: 2 servings

This dish is for people who don't have the time to cook. The flavor of the commercial sauce is enhanced by adding the juice of Kalamata olives packed in brine (contains flavor but no fat), fresh basil and a small amount of zesty Parmesan cheese. Additionally, the tomato, eggplant and chili release serotonin, so you'll feel less stressed after a long, hard day! This pasta dish is quick and easy, but tastes good enough to serve at a dinner party!

4 quarts water
4 oz. penne pasta
1 tablespoon kosher salt
1 cup Pomi's Roasted Eggplant and Tomato Sauce
1–2 tablespoons brine from a jar of Kalamata olives
4 pitted Kalamata olives, sliced
1 teaspoon red pepper flakes
2 tablespoons fresh chopped basil
2 teaspoons grated Asiagio cheese (or any sharp, good quality Italian Parmesan)

1. In a nonstick stockpot, bring water to a rolling boil, covered.
2. Add kosher salt and pasta, stir to separate pasta, and cook until al dente (8–10 minutes). Drain pasta (do not rinse pasta).
3. Put tomato sauce, Kalamata olive juice, olives and red pepper flakes in a pan. Heat until hot.
4. Add fresh basil. Remove sauce from heat and stir. (Be careful not to cook the basil—it will lose its color and flavor).
5. Add cooked pasta to hot sauce and toss until evenly coated.
6. Sprinkle with 1 teaspoon of cheese per serving.

Serving size: 6.2 ounces

CAL	FAT	PROT	CARB	FIBER	SODIUM
117	2.8 gm	4.3 gm	19.8 gm	3.1 gm	503 mg

Spaghetti Alla Sicilian

Makes: 2 servings

This pasta has only a fraction of the fat and all the flavor found in the classic Sicilian dish, pasta con le melanzan. The garlicky tomato sauce is perfumed with Italian parsley; red pepper flakes add a kiss of heat; and the anchovies impart depth to create a dish that is rich and robust. Don't let the anchovies scare you from trying this exceptional pasta—they are soaked in nonfat milk which eliminates their "fishy taste" and lend a taste and texture that is vital to the dish. One of my favorite pasta dishes.

> *4 quarts water*
> *1 tablespoon kosher salt*
> *4 ounces dried linguine*
> *2 cloves minced garlic (about 1½ teaspoons)*
> *4 anchovies, soaked in nonfat milk for 15 minutes and patted dry*
> *1 tablespoon extra-virgin olive oil*
> *2 heaping tablespoons tomato paste*
> *3 tablespoons chopped Italian flat-leaf parsley*
> *1 tablespoon Parmigiano-Reggiano cheese*
> *1 teaspoon crushed red pepper flakes*

1. Fill a large stockpot with water and bring to a rolling boil, covered.
2. Add 1 tablespoon of kosher salt to water. Add pasta to the water, stir to separate pasta, cover and cook until al dente.
3. While the pasta is cooking, pulverize the garlic with anchovies in a mortar into a thick paste.
4. Heat a heavy 8-inch nonstick pan on medium heat. Add olive oil, red pepper flakes, and cook until sizzling. Add garlic/anchovy mixture and tomato paste and stir with a whisk. Heat on medium heat until warm. Transfer sauce from pot to a small bowl.

5. Reserve ¼ cup of pasta cooking water, and drain linguine. Add pasta cooking water to the sauce and stir with a whisk until thick and creamy.

6. Transfer sauce and drained pasta back to now-empty stockpot, and toss to coat (add 2–3 tablespoons of water if dry).

7. Add parsley and toss.

8. Transfer to warm plates and top with cheese.

Serving size: 7.67 ounces

CAL	FAT	PROT	CARB	FIBER	SODIUM
311	9.7 gm	11.4 gm	44.7 gm	3.6 gm	372 mg

LINGUINE IN FRESH TOMATO SAUCE WITH FENNEL AND SALMON

Serves 4

This simple dish is a culinary fugue of flavors that packs heart-healthy phytochemicals and fish oils into each bite. The fennel gives the fresh tomato sauce a hint of sweetness, the red pepper lends a touch of heat, and the lemon zest is the perfect counterpoint flavor to accent the fish. (Do not substitute canned red salmon packed in water—the texture is too dry.)

1 tablespoon kosher salt
8 oz. dried linguine
2 teaspoons olive oil
1 teaspoon fresh, minced garlic (about 2 cloves)
1 tablespoon crushed red pepper flakes
½ teaspoon fennel seeds
2 8-oz. cans pink salmon packed in water, drained
1½ pounds ripe plum tomatoes, peeled, seeded and chopped with juices
½ teaspoon lemon zest
2 tablespoons finely chopped fresh flat-leaf Italian parsley
1 tablespoon tomato paste

1. Fill a large stockpot with 4 quarts of water, cover and bring to a rolling boil.

2. Remove pan cover, and add 1 tablespoon of kosher salt to water. Add pasta to the water and cook until al dente.

3. While pasta is cooking, pour the olive oil in a large nonstick skillet and saute the fennel seeds, red pepper flakes and garlic. Heat on medium-heat for 30 seconds, stirring constantly, until seeds release their aroma and garlic is soft. Add tomato paste and stir. Add fresh tomatoes, lemon zest and salmon (be careful not to break salmon pieces). Mix and heat. Add parsley and toss.

4. Drain spaghetti (do not rinse).

5. Add spaghetti to sauce. Gently toss to coat pasta, and cook on medium heat for several minutes until sauce thickens.

Serving size: 14.75 ounces

CAL	FAT	PROT	CARB	FIBER	SODIUM
402	10.7 gm	27.5 gm	49 gm	4.6 gm	522 mg

SHRIMP DIABLO

Makes: 1 serving

1 tablespoon kosher salt
2 ounces dried linguine
½ teaspoon olive oil
4 ounces medium shrimp (about 6 shrimp), cleaned and
    deveined with tails left on
½ teaspoon crushed red pepper flakes
2 tablespoons chopped fresh garlic
⅛ cup tequila
½ cup canned chopped tomatoes
⅛ cup Chenin Blanc wine
⅛ cup chopped Italian parsley

1. Fill a stockpot with 4 quarts of water, cover and bring to a rolling boil.

2. Remove pan cover, and add one tablespoon of kosher salt to water. Add pasta to boiling water, stir to separate pasta, and cook until al dente.

3. While pasta is cooking, heat a heavy 8-inch nonstick pan on medium heat. Mix shrimp with red pepper flakes and garlic and olive oil. Spray (1-second spray) with olive oil nonstick spray. Add shrimp to pan (shrimp should not touch each other) and sear, without moving, until bottom is lightly charred (about 20 seconds). Remove shrimp from heat and add tequila. Shake pan, and set aside. (The heat in the pan will evaporate the tequila and flavor the shrimp.) Transfer shrimp to a plate, and wipe pan clean.

4. Heat 8-inch nonstick pan on medium heat. Add tomatoes and wine, and increase the heat to medium-high. Simmer until thickened. Add shrimp and parsley and gently toss.

5. Transfer pasta to plate, and pour sauce over pasta.

CAL	FAT	PROT	CARB	FIBER	SODIUM
388	5 gm	33.1 gm	52.5 gm	4.5 gm	443 mg

MARINADES AND SAUCES

SPICY CITRUS MARINADE

This superb marinade imparts a hot, sweet and smoky flavor to grilled poultry. The acid in the citrus juice not only tenderizes leaner cuts of meats, but also imparts a sweet citrus tone to any food it touches.

> *4 cups freshly squeezed orange juice*
> *6 tablespoons freshly squeezed lime juice*
> *4 morita chilies, stems removed*
> *¼ teaspoon fresh cracked pepper*
> *4 cloves garlic, peeled*
> *1 teaspoon kosher salt*
> *juice of 1 fresh lime*
> *1 bunch cilantro, chopped*

1. Combine first 6 ingredients in a pot.
2. Bring to a boil. Reduce to a simmer for several minutes and remove from heat.
3. Remove 2 morita chilies.
4. Put mixture in a blender. Puree until smooth.
5. Add juice of 1 fresh lime and cilantro.
6. Chill overnight to let the flavors "marry."

Free Food.

Note: Foods marinated for up to 6 to 8 hours do not absorb enough sodium or oil to alter their sodium or fat content. However, longer periods of marinating will increase both the sodium and fat content of foods.

SMOKY MARINADE

If you love the smoky flavor of food cooked on an outdoor grill, this marinade is the one for you! Be sure to accurately measure the amount of liquid smoke—even a little too much will create a bitter flavor, and you will have to start over. Superb marinade for seared scallops (marinate scallops for thirty minutes before pan searing).

> 1 tablespoon soy sauce
> ½ tablespoon fresh lemon juice
> ½ tablespoon fresh lime juice
> ½ teaspoon Wright's Liquid Smoke

1. Mix all ingredients together.

Free food.

Note: Foods marinated for up to 6 to 8 hours do not absorb enough sodium or oil to alter their sodium or fat content. However, longer periods of marinating will increase both the sodium and fat content of foods.

SAVORY MEAT MARINADE

Makes: ½ cup

This marinade works wonders on lean cuts of meat, such as a London broil. The flavor of the meat is enhanced by the tannic tones of the red wine and cascabel chilies, while the acids in the balsamic vinegar, soy sauce and wine tenderize the tough fibers of the meat. You'll savor not only the rich taste but the heavenly aroma this marinade creates while the meat is grilling.

> 1 teaspoon kosher salt
> 5 cloves garlic, peeled and smashed
> ¼ cup merlot (or any full-bodied red wine)
> ¼ cup balsamic vinegar
> 1 tablespoon soy sauce
> 3–4 cascabel chilies, stems removed, soaked in hot water for
>   20 minutes until soft
> 1 teaspoon olive oil

1. Put salt and garlic in a mortar. Pulverize to a thick paste.
2. Put all ingredients in a blender.
3. Puree until smooth.

Free food.

Note: Foods marinated for up to 6 to 8 hours do not absorb enough sodium or oil to alter their sodium or fat content. However, longer periods of marinating will increase both the sodium and fat content of foods.

STEAMED VEGETABLE SAUCE

Makes: 3 servings

Although steamed vegetables are a quick and healthy side dish, they are boring. This sauce creates the smoky flavor of an outdoor grill without all the mess, or added fat. The secret of this marinade is to accurately measure out the liquid smoke—even a few extra drops will ruin it. If the marinade has a bitter flavor from too much liquid smoke, add a bit more fresh lemon juice to balance it out.

1 tablespoon sodium-reduced soy sauce
1 tablespoon fresh lemon juice
1 tablespoon Japanese seasoned rice wine vinegar
¼ teaspoon of Wright's Liquid Smoke

1. In a small bowl, add the soy sauce, lime juice, Japanese seasoned rice wine vinegar and Wright's Liquid Smoke.
2. Stir ingredients until blended.

Serving size: 1 tablespoon

CAL	FAT	PROT	CARB	FIBER	SODIUM
13	0 gm	.36 gm	2.4 gm	0 gm	371 mg

ACHIOTE CITRUS MARINADE
(FOR ROASTED POULTRY)

Makes 1½ cups

Derived from Mayan cuisine, achiote paste (recado rojo) incorporates the deep orange-red seeds of the tropical annatto tree to add both a distinctive flavor and brilliant yellow color to food. This achiote-based marinade creates a moist, savory bird with an exquisite reddish-brown skin. It's important to cook the achiote paste, which removes its chalky taste, before incorporating it into the marinade.

> 1 cup freshly squeezed orange juice (about 5 oranges)
> 4 tablespoons achiote paste
> 1 ancho chili, stem and seeds removed, cut into ¼-inch strips
> 2 jalapeno chilies, minced
> 1 jigger gold tequila
> dash cayenne
> 4 cloves garlic, minced
> ½ teaspoon kosher salt
> ½ bunch cilantro, stems and leaves, chopped
> ½ teaspoon dried Mexican oregano

1. Combine ½ cup of the orange juice with the achiote paste and stir until blended.

2. Heat the achiote-citrus mixture in an 8-inch heavy nonstick skillet pan on medium heat for several minutes until thickened. Remove and set aside.

3. Add the remainder of the ingredients to the citrus-achiote mixture.

4. Put in a blender and blend until smooth.

Free Food.

Note: Foods marinated for up to 6 to 8 hours do not absorb enough sodium or oil to alter their sodium or fat content. However, longer periods of marinating will increase both the sodium and fat content of foods.

SALSAS

Fresh Tomatillo Salsa

Makes: 4 servings

This green, tart salsa has a bracing flavor that is incomparable for cutting rich foods, such as grilled Chilean sea bass. The secret to the success of this salsa is twofold: You must first make a seasoning paste by grinding the onion, garlic and salt in a mortar, and then add the remainder of the ingredients to the paste in the given order. This technique assures that each ingredient enhances the flavor of the succeeding ones—the trick for making great salsas.

½ *white onion, minced*
2 *cloves garlic*
½ *teaspoon kosher salt*
10 *large tomatillos (about 1 pound), washed, husked and cut into*
    quarters
¼ *cup cold water*
1 *bunch fresh cilantro, stems and leaves, chopped*
1 *serrano, stemmed and minced*
1 *large jalapeno chili, stemmed and chopped*

1. Put onion, garlic and salt in a mortar. Grind to a smooth paste.

2. Put tomatillos and water in a blender and puree until smooth (you should have a thick sauce).

3. Add cilantro and puree for a few seconds until blended.

4. Add a little of the tomatillo mixture to the paste and mix to blend. Continue until all of the tomatillo mixture is blended into the paste. Remove sauce and wipe mortar.

5. Put chilies and a dash of salt in a mortar. Grind to a paste and add the tomatillo mixture to the chilies a little at a time until blended.

6. Chill for several hours to let the flavors "marry."

Kept refrigerated, this will last for 3 to 5 days.

Serving size: ½ cup

CAL	FAT	PROT	CARB	FIBER	SODIUM
55	1.4 gm	2.2 gm	10.4 gm	3.6 gm	314 mg

ROASTED SALSA VERDE

Makes: 6 servings

This recipe is a variation of the traditional Mexican sauce, salsa verde, but tastes less tart because the tomatillos are roasted, which mellows their sharp flavor. This salsa is a good choice for reserved palates, and adds mild tangy flavor to fish, chicken, potatoes or rice. The trick is to include the flavorful juices from the broiler pan, and to leave the skin on the garlic while broiling, which prevents it from burning.

> 1 pound tomatillos (approximately 10 large or 20 small),
>   husked and rinsed
> 2 jalapeno chilies, stemmed and seeds removed, minced
> ¼ large white onion
> 4 cloves garlic, skin left on
> ½ teaspoon kosher salt
> ½ cup hot water
> 1 bunch cilantro, chopped
> pinch freshly ground black pepper

1. Preheat the broiler.

2. Place the tomatillos, chilies, onion and garlic in a medium baking pan.

3. Broil, turning frequently, until all sides are lightly charred (about 15 minutes). Set aside and cool.

4. Add garlic, onion and salt to a mortar and grind to a thick paste.

5. Add chilies, tomatillos, pan juices and water (a little at a time) until a thick sauce is achieved.

6. Add cilantro.

7. Season with black pepper.

Heat level: mild

Kept refrigerated, this will last for 3 to 5 days.

Serving size: ⅓ cup

CAL	FAT	PROT	CARB	FIBER	SODIUM
39	0.9 gm	1.6 gm	7.5 gm	2.4 gm	210 mg

TIP: *The garlic and salt paste act as a seasoning, and should be used at the beginning of the process to flavor the other ingredients. If you add the paste at the end, the flavor will not be the same.*

SALSA CRUDA

Makes: 5 servings

This simple salsa is a staple in my diet. Its refreshing taste comes from contrasting fresh ingredients with bold flavors—the signature of Mexican cuisine. (Do not substitute a yellow or brown onion—you won't get the right intensity of flavor!)

5 large tomatoes, seeded and chopped (about 2 cups)
½ medium white onion, medium dice
juice of ½ freshly squeezed lemon
juice of 4 fresh limes
½ teaspoon kosher salt
4 serrano chilies, minced
½ bunch cilantro, chopped
1 teaspoon Mexican oregano, toasted
½ teaspoon olive oil

1. Put tomato, onion, lemon juice, lime juice, salt, chilies, cilantro and olive oil in a bowl and toss.
2. Take oregano and rub it between your fingers to release oil. Add to vegetable mixture and stir.
3. Chill salsa for 3 hours to let the flavors "marry."

Heat level: medium

*Kept refrigerated, this will last for 3 to 5 days.

Serving size: ½ cup

CAL	FAT	PROT	CARB	FIBER	SODIUM
34	0.8 mg	1.2 gm	7 gm	1.7 gm	248 mg

Fire-Roasted Salsa

Makes: 6 servings

This salsa has a depth of character rarely found in a simple sauce. Roasting the tomatillos, tomatoes and garlic mellows their sharp tastes and creates a rich, slightly sweet flavor and velvety texture. Do not remove the blackened skin from the vegetables—it adds a unique flavor to the salsa. This salsa is exceptional with grilled poultry, but I also love it on eggs and potatoes. (The heat level is on the hot side of "medium-hot"—reduce the crushed red pepper flakes to 2 tablespoons if you are not used to eating chilies.)

12 tomatillos, husked removed and rinsed (8 ounces)
5 roma tomatoes (24 ounces)
4 cloves garlic, skin left on
½ medium white onion, quartered
1 teaspoon kosher salt
3 tablespoons crushed red pepper flakes

1. Preheat broiler.
2. Place tomatillos, garlic and tomatoes in a 13-inch enameled roasting pan.
3. Place the roasting pan on the top rack of the oven and broil until blistered and lightly charred or blackened (about 15 minutes). Turn the vegetables and continue to broil until lightly charred (about 7 minutes). Remove roasting pan from oven, and cover with foil. Set aside and let cool for 30 minutes to allow juices to emerge.
4. Put tomatillos, tomatoes, garlic and onions, and pan juices in the blender. Blend until smooth.
5. Add salt and red pepper flakes and stir to blend.
6. Chill overnight to let the flavors "marry."

*Kept refrigerated, this will last for 5 days. Freezes well.

Serving size: ⅓ cup; 9 servings

CAL	FAT	PROT	CARB	FIBER	SODIUM
45	1.2 gm	1.6 gm	8.8 gm	2.7 gm	271 mg

CILANTRO CHUTNEY

Makes: 2 servings

This chutney has a medium heat level, and is great for cutting the rich taste of oily fish. This quick sauce has an added bonus—it doubles as a refreshing topping for potatoes. A staple in my house!

½ *teaspoon salt*
4 cloves garlic
1 large cilantro
4 serrano chilies
¼ *cup water*
2 teaspoons sugar
juice of 1 lime
1 teaspoon ground cumin

1. Pulverize salt and garlic in a mortar to form a paste.
2. Put cilantro, chilies, water, sugar, cumin and lime juice into blender and grind to form a paste.
3. Add garlic/salt mixture to cilantro mixture and blend.

Heat level: medium

*Kept refrigerated, this will last for 3 to 5 days.

Serving size: ⅓ cup

CAL	FAT	PROT	CARB	FIBER	SODIUM
36	0.5 gm	1.5 gm	7.6 gm	1.8 gm	419 mg

Red Salsa

This salsa is addictive. The secret of this salsa is using the spicy pickling juice from the jalapenos, then adding lemon juice, which acts to temper the saltiness of the brine. The pickled carrots lend a touch of sweetness and round out the taste. This salsa has a medium heat level, and a flavor that really picks up the taste of poultry, fish or soft tacos. You'll get the best results if you use homemade pickled chilies from a Latin market, or canned pickled jalapenos from Mexico.

2 large tomatoes, peeled, seeded and chopped
5 pickled jalapenos, chopped
4 pickled carrot slices
2 tablespoons chopped white onion
½ cup vinegar from pickled jalapenos
juice of 1½ lemons
¼ teaspoon Mexican oregano, toasted
¼ teaspoon salt

1. Put tomatoes, chilies, carrots, onion and pickling juice in a blender and blend.
2. Add lemon juice, oregano and salt to taste.

Heat level: medium hot

*Kept refrigerated, this will last for 3 to 5 days.

Serving size: ½ cup

CAL	FAT	PROT	CARB	FIBER	SODIUM
66	0.6 gm	1.8 gm	13.5 gm	3.3 gm	523 mg

TIP: If you don't have time to peel the tomatoes by blanching the skin, use this handy technique. Cut a tomato in half and scoop out the seeds. Place the cut side of the tomato against the largest opening of a food grater and gently rub the tomato until you reach the skin. Discard the skin.

Salsa Rojo

Makes: 4 servings

The secret ingredient in this salsa is cloves, which impart a haunting note. This salsa needs to be chilled overnight to fully develop its complex flavor. An exquisite salsa for soft chicken tacos and burritos. Freezes well.

2 guajillo chilies, stems removed
1 pound of tomatillos, husks removed and rinsed (about 20 tomatillos)
15 arbol chilies, toasted
1 large clove garlic
3 black peppercorns
½ teaspoon ground cumin
2 whole cloves
½ teaspoon kosher salt

1. In a 2-quart pot, put the guajillo chilies and tomatillos. Add enough water to just cover chilies and tomatillos (about 3 cups).
2. Cook until tomatillos are soft. Remove from heat and cool.
3. Put chilies and tomatillos in a blender, and blend until smooth.
4. Add the remainder of the ingredients, and blend until smooth.
5. Chill overnight to let the flavors "marry."

Heat level: medium hot

Kept refrigerated, this will last for 5 to 7 days. Freezes well.

Serving size: ⅓ cup

CAL	FAT	PROT	CARB	FIBER	SODIUM
63	1.4 gm	2.3 gm	33 gm	3.5 gm	298 mg

Leaving the skin on the garlic while roasting not only prevents it from burning but creates a smoky flavor. You'll get the best results if you use ripe tomatoes. Where the jalapenos have been grown determines the heat level of this salsa.

ROASTED JALAPENO SALSA

Makes: 3 servings

3 jalapeno chilies
5 large plum tomatoes
1 clove garlic (leave skin on)
½ teaspoon salt

1. Heat a heavy cast iron skillet, comal (Mexican pan available from specialty stores) or griddle on medium heat until hot. Dry roast chilies, tomatoes and garlic until slightly charred on all sides. (As one side of vegetable blackens, turn the vegetable with tongs until all the sides are charred and blistered.)

2. Remove chili stems and garlic skin. Coarsely chop the roasted chilies.

3. Put chilies, tomatoes, garlic and salt in a blender on medium speed until smooth.

4. Add salt and stir to blend.

5. Chill salsa overnight to let flavors "marry."

Heat level: medium hot

Kept refrigerated, this will last for 5 to 7 days. Freezes well.

Serving size: ⅓ cup

CAL	FAT	PROT	CARB	FIBER	SODIUM
20	0.3 gm	0.8 gm	4.2 gm	1.2 gm	394 mg

ROASTED SERRANO SALSA

Makes: 3 servings

This salsa is hot—use only if you are used to chilies.

12 serrano chilies
3 large tomatoes
1 clove garlic
2 arbol chilies, toasted
salt to taste

1. Put chilies and tomatoes in a packet of foil.

2. Put aluminum foil package over a gas burner on medium heat until soft.

3. Remove chilies and tomatoes, and place in a blender. Add one clove of garlic and blend until smooth.

Heat level: hot

Kept refrigerated, this will last for 5 to 7 days. Freezes well.

Serving size: ⅓ cup

CAL	FAT	PROT	CARB	FIBER	SODIUM
55	0.9 gm	2.3 gm	11.9 gm	3.3 gm	115 mg

AVOCADO SALSA

Makes: 11 servings

While guacamole is a good source of healthy monounsaturated fat, eating too much of this luscious sensual treat will pack on the pounds. This recipe delivers all the rich flavors of a zesty guacamole at only 1.8 grams of fat per serving! The secret is using a small amount of California Hass (thick, bumpy, black-skinned) avocado, which has a richer flavor than their thin-skinned, watery Florida cousins. Also limit your portion to 2 tablespoons (⅛ cup) to keep the fat grams low. This salsa doubles as a salad dressing, and freezes well. (Pour extra salsa into an ice cube tray, and cover with plastic wrap. Each cube holds 2 tablespoons, which portion controls the avocado salsa to just the right amount.)

> 1 small, ripe Hass avocado, peeled and seeded (4½ ounces)
> 1 cup water
> juice of ½ lemon (1½ tablespoons)
> 2 serrano chilies, chopped
> ¼ cup fresh cilantro, loosely packed
> ½ teaspoon kosher salt

1. Put avocado and water in a blender and blend until smooth.
2. Put the remainder of the ingredients in a blender and blend until smooth.

Heat level: mild

Kept refrigerated, this will last for 3 to 5 days.

Serving size: ⅛ cup

CAL	FAT	PROT	CARB	FIBER	SODIUM
20	1.8 gm	0.3 gm	1.2 gm	0.7 gm	109 mg

SEASONING
BLENDS

SMOKY PASADO CHILI SEASONING BLEND

Makes: 6 servings

This savory seasoning blend transforms bland cottage cheese into something you'll *want* to eat. Moreover, it provides a lot less sodium than salt, which packs a whopping 1,172 mg per ½ teaspoon! Doubles as a dry spice-rub for meat, poultry and fish, and its slightly sweet, smoky flavor works wonders on sliced fresh tomatoes.

> 2 tablespoons pasado chili powder (grind
>   3 to 4 dried pasado chilies; remove stems)
> ¼ teaspoon dried garlic granules
> ¼ teaspoon onion powder
> ¼ teaspoon kosher salt
> ¼ teaspoon black pepper

1. Blend all the ingredients in a coffee grinder to form a seasoning blend.

TIP: To get an even consistency, grind the chilies and spices for 10 seconds, then stop. Shake the coffee grinder and regrind. Repeat this step several times.

Serving size: ½ teaspoon

CAL	FAT	PROT	CARB	FIBER	SODIUM
7	0.3 gm	0.3 gm	1.2 gm	0.5 gm	98 mg

Chili Pepper Diet Recado (Dry)

Makes 1 cup

In Mexico, markets sell a variety of prepared wet and dry seasonings—recado, adobo, puchero, mechado, chilaquil, salpimentado and alcarrado—for enhancing the flavor of foods. This recipe is a healthier (less salt and fat) version of the traditional Yucatan dry spice rub, recado, which is used to both color and flavor meat, fish, poultry and corn before grilling. This exceptional seasoning mixture imparts robust, smoky flavors to poultry, meat, steamed vegetables, low-fat cottage cheese and low-fat mayonnaise.

> 5 ancho chilies, stems and seeds removed
> 1 morita chili, stem removed
> 4 chipolte chilies, stems removed
> ½ cup dried onion
> ¼ cup dried Mexican oregano
> 3 tablespoons kosher salt
> 25 cloves fresh garlic, minced (approximately
>   1 head of garlic)

1. Cut ancho chilies the length of one side and lay out flat. Stack several flattened ancho chilies on top of each other and roll into cylinder (the shape of a cigarette). Cut chilies into ¼-inch strips with a knife or scissors. Cut whole morita and chipotle into ¼-inch strips.

2. Heat a heavy nonstick skillet until hot. Spray with a vegetable spray (twice) and add ancho chilies. Spray chilies with vegetable spray (once) and toast until fragrant (be careful not to burn the chilies or they will take on a bitter taste). Remove toasted chilies and wipe pan clean. Repeat process with the remaining chilies. Set aside to cool.

3. Put onion, chilies and oregano into a 1-cup blender container or attachment. Grind mixture until the texture of coarse sand is achieved.

4. Add garlic and pulse until the spice mixture has the consistency of wet sand.

5. Cover and store recado in the refrigerator.

TIP: If the recado gets sticky, spread the spice rub into a thin layer on a baking sheet and heat in the oven at 200° for 1 hour. Regrind spice rub before using.

*Kept refrigerated, this will last 1 month.

Serving size: 1 tablespoon

CAL	FAT	PROT	CARB	FIBER	SODIUM
4	0	0.1 gm	0.8 gm	0.1 gm	163 mg

SMOKY RECADO PASTE

Although this recado paste contains basically the same ingredients as the spice rub, it has a more complex taste because the ingredients are first roasted, and then combined in a mortar to create a flavorful paste. Makes a great seasoning for broiled fish, roasted poultry and steamed brown rice! Traditionally, a spicy salsa is served with grilled recado-seasoned foods to balance their smoky, rich flavor.

> 5 ancho chilies, stems and seeds removed
> 1 morita chili, stem removed
> 4 chipotle chilies, stems removed
> 1 cup chopped white onion, dry roasted till lightly charred and soft
> ¼ cup kosher salt
> ¼ cup dried, toasted Mexican oregano
> 25 cloves fresh garlic, minced (approximately 1 head of garlic)
> 2 plum tomatoes, chopped and dry roasted until lightly charred
> 1 teaspoon corn oil

1. Cut ancho chilies the length of one side and lay out flat. Stack several flattened ancho chilies on top of each other and roll into cylinder (the shape of a cigarette). Cut chilies into ¼-inch strips with a knife or scissors. Cut morita and chipotle chilies into ¼-inch strips.

2. Heat a heavy medium nonstick pan until hot. Spray with a vegetable spray (twice) and add ancho chilies. Spray top of chilies with vegetable spray (once) and toast until fragrant (be careful not to burn the chilies or they will take on a bitter taste). Remove toasted chilies and wipe pan clean. Repeat process with the remaining chilies. Set aside to cool.

3. Put onion, chilies, salt and oregano into a 1-cup blender container or attachment. Grind until the texture of coarse sand is achieved.

4. Add garlic and salt. Pulse until the spice mixture has the consistency of wet sand.

5. Add tomatoes and grind to a thick paste.

6. Add oil and stir to blend.

Kept refrigerated, this will last 2 weeks.

Serving size: 1 teaspoon

CAL	FAT	PROT	CARB	FIBER	SODIUM
4	0 gm	0.1 gm	0.8 gm	0.1 gm	163 mg

TIP: *Use pastes, rather than dry spice rubs, when using dry-heat cooking methods to prepare low-fat foods. Their moisture helps to prevent the food from drying out during the cooking process.*

ACHIOTE PASTE (RECADO ROJO)

Makes: ⅓ cup

Derived from Mayan cuisine, achiote paste incorporates the deep orange-red seeds of the tropical annatto tree. This annatto-based recado is used to add both a distinctive flavor and brilliant yellow color to marinades, sauces and poultry dishes.

>1 tablespoon annatto seeds
>¼ teaspoon cumin seeds, toasted
>¼ teaspoon dried Mexican oregano, lightly toasted
>8 black peppercorns
>½ teaspoon allspice
>1 clove
>4 piquin chilies (or any small, hot, dried chili)
>½ teaspoon kosher salt
>4 cloves garlic, smashed
>¼ cup freshly squeezed orange juice mixed with 1 tablespoon
>   freshly squeezed grapefruit juice

1. Put annatto seeds, cumin seeds, oregano, peppercorns, allspice, clove and chili in a coffee grinder and grind to a powder.

2. Pulverize garlic and salt in a mortar or molcajete (Mexican stone mortar) into a smooth paste.

3. Add the ground spice mixture to the garlic paste and mix to blend.

4. Add citrus juices, stirring, until a thick paste is achieved.

5. Put the achiote paste in a glass container (achiote will stain plastic), cover and refrigerate.

Kept refrigerated, this will last 3 to 4 days.

Serving size: 1 tablespoon

CAL	FAT	PROT	CARB	FIBER	SODIUM
17	0.3 gm	0.5 gm	3.6 gm	0.5 gm	236 mg

DESSERTS

SPICY GINGERED PEARS
WITH LEMON CREAM

Makes: 2 servings

This fruit dessert tastes so elegant, it could be served in a fine French restaurant. The ginger, pineapple juice and molasses create a rich, sweet syrup that enhances the delicate flavor of the pears. Top with a generous dollop of lemon cream, and you won't miss the artery-clogging creme brulee! Be sure to reduce the fruit juice to a syrup to get the right intensity of flavor. This dish can be served warm or chilled.

> 1 cup pineapple juice
> 1 tablespoon dark molasses
> 1 pear, peeled, cored and sliced in half
> ½ teaspoon fresh minced ginger
> ½ teaspoon freshly squeezed lemon juice
> 2 pinches cayenne chili powder

1. Put all ingredients in a pot.
2. Simmer pear halves and sauce on medium-low heat until pears are tender but not mushy (about 3 to 4 minutes). Remove pears and transfer to a plate.
3. Continue cooking juice until a thick syrup is achieved (about 4 minutes more, you should reduce the juice to ¼ cup).
4. Strain syrup and let cool.
5. Place half a poached pear on a plate and pour sauce around pear.
6. Top with 1 tablespoon lemon cream.

Lemon Cream

¼ cup ReddiWhip Fat-Free Dairy Topping
2 teaspoons freshly squeezed lemon juice

1. Gently fold the lemon juice into the ReddiWhip until the consistency of a thick cream.

2. Drizzle cream over pears.

Serving size: ½ poached pear, 2 tablespoons syrup, 1 tablespoon of lemon cream

CAL	FAT	PROT	CARB	FIBER	SODIUM
159	0.5 gm	0.8 gm	39.4 gm	2.4 gm	8 gm

Strawberry Gelato

Makes: 4 servings

Rich flavors and luscious textures don't always come from high-fat ingredients. Combining frosty evaporated milk and frozen fruit creates a sensuous dessert that rivals ice cream. This dessert tastes best when served right after preparation—do not freeze. I love this recipe—it saves me a trip to the frozen yogurt shop when I get a craving for something rich, cold and creamy.

1 large ripe banana, cut in 1-inch chunks and frozen (about 1 cup)
1 cup frozen strawberries, cut in 1-inch chunks
1 cup nonfat evaporated milk, chilled in freezer for 25 minutes

1. Remove frozen fruit from freezer for 10 minutes.
2. Place bananas in blender and process at medium speed until pureed (bananas should be thick and slightly chunky). Add strawberries, and repeat process with second batch of frozen fruit.
3. In a slow steady stream, add chilled nonfat milk to fruit mixture while blender is running on medium speed until you get a thick, creamy consistency.
4. Serve.

Serving size: ½ cup

CAL	FAT	PROT	CARB	FIBER	SODIUM
104	0.4 gm	5.4 gm	21.1 gm	2.3 gm	75 mg

WHERE TO FIND CHILI PRODUCTS

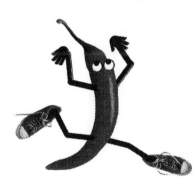

Nancy's Healthy Kitchen Lite Blue Cheese Dressing
Chris Kay, Inc.
(818) 341-7661

Will ship product via FedEx (overnight).

If you *love* blue cheese dressing, put a check in the mail for this product! This salad dressing *really* does taste like the real thing.

The Chili Guy
(800) 869-9218

Great source for hard-to-get New Mexican and South American dried chilies. Primarily services restaurant trade, but will ship to home consumers in large quantities (five to twenty-five pounds). Ask to have a current price guide faxed before ordering chilies.

Monterrey Foods

www.monterreyfoodproducts.com

Excellent source for a variety of dried chilies and Mexican food products. Will ship chilies in small quantities, and prices are *very* reasonable. Request a product list for current products and prices.

Uncle Bum's Hot Jamaican Marinade

Uncle Bum's

(800) 486-2867

This product is sold primarily to hotels and restaurants, and is getting more difficult to find in markets. However, the manufacturer will ship twelve (12-oz.) jars for $41.00 (this price includes shipping). At $3.41 per bottle, this price is *below* retail!

BIBLIOGRAPHY

Why Diets Fail

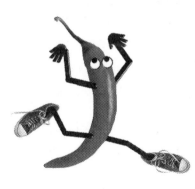

J. Jeppesen et al., "Effects of low-fat diet, high-carbohydrate diets on risk factors for ischemic heart disease in postmenopausal women," Am J Clin Nutr (1997), 65:1027–33.

J. Dengel et al., "Effect of an American Heart Association diet, with or without weight loss, in lipids in obese middle-aged and older men," Am J Clin Nutr (1995), 62:715–21.

R. Mattes, "Fat preference and adherence to a reduced-fat diet," Am J Clin Nutr (1994), 57:373–81.

JE Blundell et al., "Mechanisms of appetite control and their abnormalities in obese patients," Horm Res (1993), 39(suppl 3):72–76.

A Kristal et al., "Long-term maintenance of a low-fat diet: Durability of fat-related dietary habits in the Women's Health Trial," J Am Diet Ass (1992 May), 92(5):553–59.

C Henry et al., "Effect of spiced food on matabolic rate," Hom Nutr Clin Nutr (1986), 40:165–8.

E Doucet et al., "Food intake, energy balance and body weight control," Env J Clin Nutr, (Dec 1997), 51 (12):846–55.

Yoshioka et al., "Effects of red pepper added to high-fat diet and high-carbohydrate meals on energy metabolism and substrate utilization in Japanese women," Brit J Nutr, (Dec 1998), 80(16):503–10.

DG Schlundt et al., "A behavioral taxonomy of obese female participants in a weight-loss program," Am J Clin Nutr (1991 May), 53(5):1151–8.

A Trunswell, "Practical and realistic approaches to healthier diet modifications," Am J Clin Nutr (1998), 67(suppl):583S–90S.

J Fernstrom and G Miller, Appetite and Weight Regulation: Sugar, Fat and Macronutrient Substitutes, CRC Press, Boca Raton, Florida, 1994.

U Erasmus, Fats that Heal, Fats that Kill, Canada: Alive Books, 1995.

M Katan, "High oil compared to low-fat, high-carbohydrate diets in the prevention of ischemic heart disease," Am J Clin Nutr (1997), 66(suppl): 974s–9s.

A Conner et al., "Are fish oils beneficial in the prevention and treatment of coronary artery disease?", Am J Clin Nutr (1997), 66(suppl): 1020s–31s.

T Szabo et al., "Pharmocological characterization of the vanilloid receptor located in the brain," Molecular Brain Research, 98(2002):51–57.

The Chili Connection

E Scharrer, et al., "Control of food intake by fatty acid oxidation," Am J H Physiol (1986), 250:R1003.

S Ritter, et al., "Vagal sensory neurons are required for lipoprivic but not glucoprivic feeding in rats," Am J Physiol (1990):258, R1395.

S Ritter et al., "Capsaicin abolishes liporivic but not glucoprivic feeding in rats," Am J Physiol (1989):R1232.

P Holzer, et al., "Capsaicin: cellular targets, mechanisms of action, and selectivity for thin sensory neurons," Pharm Rev (1991), 43:143.

N Calingasan, et al., "Presence of galalnin in rat vagal sensory neurons: an immunohistochemical and situ hybridization study," J Autonom Nerv Syst (1992), 40:229.

N Calingsan, et al., "Blockade of fatty acid oxidation increases the number vagal sensory neurons containing galalin mRNA and hnRNA, Soc Neurosci, Abstr. (1992), 18:896.

M Koltzenburg, "The changing sensitivity in the life of the nociceptor," Pain (1999 Aug), Suppl 6:S93–102.

AL Krogstad et al., "Capsaicin treatment in histamine release and perfusion changes in psoriatic skin," Brit J Derm (1994 Jul), 141(1):87–93.

K Platel et al. "Influence of dietary spices and their active principles on pancreatic digestive enzymes in albino rats," Nahrung (2000 Feb), 44(1):42–6.

T Samasura et al., "Peripheral and central actions of capsaicin and vanilloid receptor," Jpn. J Pharm (1999 Aug), 80(4):275–80.

TK Yun et al., "Update from Asia on cancer chemoprevention," Annuals of the New York Academy of Sciences (1999), 899:157–92.

YJ Surh et al., "Inhibitory effects of curcumin and capsaicin on phorbol ester-induced activation of eukaryotic transcription factors, NF-kappaB and Ap-1," Biofactors (2000), 12(1–4):107–12.

YJ Surh et al., Chemoprotective properties of some pungent ingredients present in red pepper and ginger," Mutation Research (1998),40:259–67.

RW Gear et al., "Pain-induced analgesia mediated by mesolimbic reward circuits, " J Neuro (1999 Aug 15), 19(16):7175–81.

E Scharrer, "Control of food intake by fatty acid oxidation and ketogenesis," Nutrition (1999 Sept), 15(9):704–14.

B Joe et al., "Dietary n-3 fatty acids, curcumin and capsaicin lower the release of lysosomal enzymes in rat peritoneal macrophages," Molecular and Cellular Biochemistry (2000), 203:153–61.

A Saito et al., "Effects of capsaicin on serum triglycerides and free fatty acid in olive oil treated rats," International Journal for Vitamin and Nutritional Research (1999 Sept), 69(5):33.

T Biro et al., "Specific vanilloid responses in C6 rat glioma cells," Mol Brain Res (1998b), 56:89–98.

T Biro et al., "Characterization of functional vanilloid receptors expressed in mast cells," Blood (1998 a), 91:1332–40.

SH Buck et al., "The neuropharmacology of capsaicin: A review of some recent observations," Pharmocol Rev (1986), 38:179–226

MJ Caterina et al., " The capsaicin receptor: A heat-activated ion channel in the pain pathway," Nature (1997), 389:816–24.

MB Chancellor, Editorial: "Should we be using chili pepper extracts to treat the overactive bladder?" J Urol (1997), 158:2097.

DeGrout, "A neurologic basis for the overactive bladder," Urology (1997), 50 (Suppl 6A):36–52.

F Cruz, "Densensitization of the bladder sensory fibers by intravesical capsaicin or capsaicin analogs. A new strategy for the treatment of urge incontinence in patients with spinal destrusor hyperfelxia or bladder hypersensitivity disorders," Int Urogynecol J (1998), 9:214–29.

F Cruz et al., "Densensitization of bladder sensory fibers by intravesical capsaicin has long-lasting clinical and urodynamic effects in patients with hyperactive or hypersensitive dysfunction," J Urol (1997b), 157:585–89.

T. Sasamura, "Existence of capsaicin-sensitive glutamatergic terminals in rat hypothalmus," Neuroreport (1998), 9:2045–2048.

G. Partsch, "Capsaicin stimulates the migration of human polymorphonuclear cells (PMN) in vitro," Life Sciences (1993), 53:PL309–PL314.

J. Porszasz, "Cardiovascular and respiratory effects of capsaicin," Acta Physiol Hung (1955), 8:61–76.

G. Makara et al., "Circulatory and respiratory responses to capsaicin, 5-dyroxytryptamine in rats pretreated with capsaicin," Arch Int Pharmacodyn Ther (1967), 170:39–45.

A. Szallasi et al., "Characterization by [3H] resiniferatoxin of a human vanilliod (capsaicin) receptor in post-mortem spinal cord," Neurosci Lett (1994), 165:101–4.

BH Marciniak et al., "Adverse consequences of capsaicin exposure in health care workers," J AM Geriatr Soc (1995), 43:1181–2.

GR Lewin et al., "Nerve growth factor and nociception," Trends Neurosci (1993), 16:353–59.

K Lim et al., "Dietary red pepper ingestion increases carbohydrate oxidation at rest and during exercise in runners," Med Sci Sports Exerc (1997), 29:355–61.

JM Lundberg et al., "Tachykinins, sensory nerves and asthma—an overview," Can J Physiol Pharmacol (1995), 73:908–14.

P Stjarneet et al., "Capsaicin desensitization of the nasal mucosa reduces symptoms upon allergen challenge in patients with allergic rhinitis," Acta Otolaryngol (1998), 118:235–39.

F Filiaciet et al., "Local treatment of nasal polyposis with capsaicin: Preliminary findings," Allergol Immunopathol (1996), 24:13–18.

F Sicuteri et al., "Beneficial effect of capsaicin application to the nasal mucosoa in cluster headaches," Clinic J Pain (1989), 5:49–53.

DR Marks et al., "A double-blind, placebo-controlled trial of intranasal capsaicin in cluster headache," Cephalagia (1993), 13:114–6.

J Wallengren et al., "Treatment of notalgia paresthetica with topical capsaicin," J Am Acad Dermatol (1991), 24:286–8.

JE Bernstein et al., "Capsaicin in dermatologic diseases," Semin Dermatol (1988), 7:304–9.

CN Ellis et al., "A double-blind evaluation of topical capsaicin in puritic psoriasis," J Am Acad Dermatol (1993), 29:438–42.

DL Breneman et al., "Topical capsaicin for treatment of hemodialysis-related pruritus," J Am Acad Dermatol (1992), 26:91–94.

KM Basha et al., "Capsaicin: A therapeutic option for painful diabetic polyneuropathy," Henry Ford Hosp Med J (1991), 39:138–40.

NM Scheffler et al., "Treatment of painful diabetic neuropathy with capsaicin," J Am Podiatr Med Assoc (1991), 81:288–293.

PA Low et al., "Double-blind, placebo-controlled study of the application of capsaicin cream in chronic distal painful polyneuropathy," Pain (1995), 62:163–8.

D Dini et al., "Treatment of the postmastectomy pain syndrome with topical capsaicin," Pain (1993), 54:223–6.

GM McCarthy et al., "Effect of topical capsaicin in the therapy of painful arthritis of the hands," J Rheumatol (1992), 19:604–7.

R Gonzalez et al., "Effects of capsaicin-containing red pepper sauce suspension on upper gastrointestinal motility in healthy human beings," Dig Sis Sci (1998), 43:1165–71.

H Sasaki et al., "New strategies for aspiration pneumonia," Intern Med (1997), 36:851–5.

CJK Henry et al., "Effect of spiced food on metabolic rate," Hum Nutr Clin Nutr (1986), 40:165–68.

D Cameron-Smith et al., "Capsaicin and dihydrocapaicin stimulate oxygen consumption in perfused rat hindlimb," Int J Obes (1990), 4:259–70.

E Doucet et al., "Food intake, energy balance and body weight control," Eur J Clin Nutr (1997), 51:846–55.

T Kawadaet et al., "Capsaicin-induced beta-adrenergic action on energy metabolism in rats: Influence of capsaicin on oxygen consumption, the respiratory quotient, and substrate utilization," Proc Soc Exp Biol Med (1986), 183:250–56.

T Watanabe et al., "Capsaicin, a pungent principle of hot pepper, evokes catecholamine secretion from the adrenal medulla of anesthetized rats," Biochem Biophys Res Commun (1987), 142:259–64.

PLR Andrew et al., "Resiniferatoxin, an ultra potent capsaicin analogue, has anitemetic properties in the ferret," Neuropharmacology (1993), 32:799–806.

A Szallasi, "Vanilloid (capsaicin) receptors in the rat: Distribution the brain, regional differences the spinal cord, axonal transport to the periphery, and depletion by systemic vanilliod treatment," Brain Res (1995), 703: 175–83.

N Matsuki et al., "Role of substance P in emesis," Folia Pharmacol Jpn (1996), 108:133–38.

RW Gear, et al., "Pain-induced analgesia mediated by mesolimbic reward circuits," J Neuro (1999 Aug 15), 19(16):7175.

Y Shirosita et al., "Capsaicin in the 4th ventricle abolishes retching and transmission of emeteic vagal efferents to the solitary nucleus neurons," Eur J Pharmacol (1997), 339:183–92.

NL Jones et al., "Capsaicin as an inhibitor of the gastric pathogen Helicobacter pylori," FEMS Microbiol Lett (1997), 146:223–27.

E Dourin, " Helicobacter pylori: novel therapies," Can J Gastro (1999 Sept), 13(7):581–3.

RW Brusker, "Toxicologic evaluation of pepper spray as a possible weapon for the Dutch police force: risk assessment and efficiency," Amer J of Forensic Med and Path (1998 Dec), 19(4):309–

S Basak et al., "Effects of capsaicin pre-treatment in experimentally-induced secretory otitis media," J Laryn and Otology (1999 Feb), 113(2):114–7.

P Bjorntrop, "Body Fat Distribution, Insulin Resistance, and Metabolic Diseases," Nutrition (1997), 13(a):795–803.

P Bjorntorp, "Obesity and Cortisol," Nutrition (2000), 16(10):924–35.

ES Epel, "Stress and Body Shape: stress-induced cortisol secretion is consistently greater among women with central fat," Psychosom Med (2000 Sept-Oct), 62(5):623–32.

P Bjorntorp, "Stress and Cardiovascular Disease," Acta Physiol Scand Suppl (1997), 640:144–8.

P Bjorntorp, "Hypothalmbic arousal, insulin resistance and Type 2, diabetes mellitus," Diabet Med (1999 May), 16(5):373–83.

P Bjorntorp, "Neuroendocrine perturbations as a cause of insulin resistance," Diabetes Metab Res Rev (1999 Nov-Dec), 15(6):427–41.

V Vicennati et al., "Abnormalities of the hypothalamic-pituitary-adrenal axis in nondepressed women with abdominal obesity and relations with insulin resistance: evidence for a central and a peripheral alteration," J Clin Endocrinol Metab (2000 Nov), 85(11):4093–8.

R Rosmond et al., "The role of antidepressants in the treatment of abdominal obesity," Med Hypotheses (2000 Jun), 54(6):990–4.

KN Frayn, "Visceral fat and insulin resistance—causative or correlative?" Br J Nutr (2000 Mar), 83 Suppl. 1:S71–7.

P Bjorntorp, "Endocrine abnormalities of obesity," Metabolism (1995 Sep), 44(9)suppl. 3:21–3.

S Koopmans, "Neonatal de-afferenation of capsaicin-sensitive sensory nerves increases in vivo insulin sensitivity in conscious adult rats," Diabetologia (1998), 41:813–20.

E Guillot et al., "Involvement of capsaicin-sensitive nerves in the regulation of glucose tolerance in diabetic rats," Life Sciences (1996), 59(12):969–77.

V Coiro et al., "Neuroendocrinology," (1992), 56:459–63.

JA Negulesco et al., "Capsaicin lowers plasma cholesterol and triglycerides of lagomorphs," Arterv (1985)m 12L30–11.

JA Negulesco et al., "Effects of pure capsaicinoids (capsaicin and dihydrocapsaicin) on plasma lipid and lipoprotein concentrations of turkey poulds," Atherosclerosis (1987 Apr), 64 (2–3):85–90.

R Buffensteine, et al., "Food intake and the menstrual cycle: a retrospective analysis with implication for appetite research," Physiol Behav (1995), 58:1067–1077.

K Bruinsma, et al., "Chocolate: food or drug?" J Am Diet Assoc. (1999), 99:1249–1256.

N Yamaguchi et al., "Sympathoadrenal system in neuroendocrine control of glucose: mechanisms involved in the liver, pancreas, and adrenal gland under hemorrhagic stress and hypoglycemic stress," Can J Physiol Pharmacol (1992 Feb), 70:167–206.

P Holzer, "Capsaicin: cellular targets, mechanisms of action, and selectivity for thin sensory neurons," Pharmcol Rev (1991), 43:143–201.

XF Zhou et al., "Capsaicin-sensitive nerves are required for glucostatsis but not for catecholamine output during hypoglycemia in rats," Am J Physiol (1990), 258:E212–E9.

S Karlsson et al., "Involvement of capsaicin-sensitive nerves in regulation of insulin secretion and glucose tolerance in conscious mice," Am J Physiol (1994), 267:R1071–R77.

B Ahren et al., "Neuropeptidergic versus cholinergic and adrenegic regulation of islet hormone secretion," Diabetologia (1986), 29:827–36.

AG Dulloo, "Spicing fat for combustion," Br J Nutr (1998 Dec), 80(6):493–4.

Z Tang et al., "Involvement of capsaicin-sensitive sensory nerves in early protection and delayed cardioprotection induced by a brief ischaemia of the small intestine," Naunyn-Schmiedeberg's Archives of Pharmacology (1999), 359(3):234–47.

R Lee, "The effects of acute moderate exercise on serum lipids and lipoproteins in mildly obese women," Inter J Sports Med (1991 Dec), 12(6):537–42.

CY Bae et al., "A clinical trail of the American Heart Association step one diet for the treatment of hypercholesterolemia," J Fam Prac (1991 Sept), 33(3):249–54.

E Douchet, et al., "Appetite after weight loss by energy restriction and a low-fat diet-exercise follow-up," Int Journ of Obesity and Met Disorders (2000 Jul), 24(7):906–14.

J Marniemi et al., "Long-term effects of lipid metabolism of weight reduction on lacovegetarian and mixed diets," Int J Obes (1990 Feb 14), 2:113–25.

R Leenen et al., "Relative effects of weight loss and dietary fat modification on serum lipid levels in the dietary treatment of obesity," J of Lipid Res (1993)Dec, 34(12):2183–91.

CJ Billingtonet et al., "Neuropeptide Y in hypothalamic paraventicular nulceus: a center coordinating energy metabolism," Am J Phy (1994 Jun), 6(2):R1765–70.

LP Lowell et al., "Development of obesity in transgenic mice after genetic ablation of brown adipose tissue," Nature (1993 Dec), 366(6457):740–2.

GA Grey et al., "Food intake, sympathetic activity, and adrenal steriods," Brain Res Bull (1993), 32(5):537–41.

NS Govindarajan et al. "Capsicum—production, pharmacology, nutrition, and quality. Part V. Impact on physiology, pungency, pain, and desensitization sequences," Crit Rev in Food Sci and Nutr, (1991), 29(6):435–74.

MB Katan, "High-oil compared with low-fat, high carbohydrate diets in the prevention of ischemic heart disease," Am J Clin Nutr (1997), 66(suppl.):974S–9S.

C Gartner, "Lycopene is more bioavailable from tomato paste than from fresh tomatoes," Am J Clin Nutr (1997), 66:116–22.

B Nicklas et al., "Effects of an American Heart Association diet and weight loss on lipoprotein lipids in obese, postmenopausal women," J Clin Nutr (1997) 66:853–9.

A Ascherio et al., "Health effects of trans fatty acids," Am J Clin Nutr (1997), 66(suppl):1006S–10S.

M Oliver, "It is more important to increase the intake of unsaturated fats than to decrease the intake of saturated fats: evidence from clinical trials relating to ischemic heart disease," Am J Clin Nutr (1997), 66(suppl): 980S–6S.

M Klem et al., " A descriptive study of individuals successful at long-term maintenance of substantial weight loss," Am J Clin Nutr (1997), 66:239–46.

W Robbins, "Clinical Application of Capsaicinoids," The Clinical Journal of Pain (2000), 16:S86–S89.

A Szallasi et al., "Vanilloid (Capsaicin) Receptors and Mechanisms," Phar Rev (1999 Jun), 51(2):159–212.

L Kiwon, et al., "Dietary red pepper ingestion increases carbohydrate oxidation at rest and during exercise in runners," Med and Science in Sports and Exer (1997), 335–361.

Not All Chilies Are Created Equal

CJ Henry, et al., "Effect of spiced food on metabolic rate," Hum Clin Nutr (1986), 40:165–168.

W Robbins, "Clinical Application of Capsaicinoids," The Clinical Journal of Pain (2000), 16:S86–S89.

New Mexico State University Department of Agronomy and Horticulture Chilies.

American Spice Trade Association (ASTA Information Bureau).

D Dewitt, The Chili Pepper Encyclopedia, New York: Morrow, 1999.

J Andrews, Red Hot Chilies, New York: Macmillan, 1993.

The Chili Pepper Diet

S Kleiner, "Water: An essential but overlooked nutrient," J Amer Diet Assoc (1999 Feb), 99(2):200–6.

K Bruinsma et al., "Chocolate: Food or Drug?" J Am Diet Assoc (1999), 99:1249–56.

PC Zemel et al., "Regulation of adiposity by dietary calcium," FASEB J(2000), 14:1132–38.

KM Davies et al., "Calcium intake and body weight," Journal of Clinical Endocrinology & Metabolism (2000), 85(12):4635–9.

PC Zemel et al., "Increasing dietary calcium and dairy product consumption reduces the relative risk of obesity in humans," Obesity Res (2000), 8:118.

Alert on Lead in Calcium, Los Angeles Times, Oct. 2000 (Health Section) [The authors' results appeared in the Sep 20 issue of the Journal of the American Medical Association].

W Leary, "A Recipe for Weight Gain: Adding Alcohol to Fatty Food," The New York Times (Health Section), Sep 6, 1995.

GA Coldita et al., "Alcohol intake in relation to diet and obesity in women and men," Am J Clin Nut (1991 July), 54(1):49–55.

CR Markus et al., "Carbohydrate intake improves cognitive performance of stress-prone individuals under controllable laboratory stress," Brit J Nutr (1999), 82:457–67.

D Allison et al., "Estimated intakes of trans fats and other fatty acids in the US population," Research (1999 Feb), 99(2): 166–74.

ADA Reports, "Position of the American Dietetic Association: Functional Foods," J ADA Assoc (1999 October), 99(10):1278–85.

TA Mori et al., "Effects of varying dietary fat, fish and fish oils on blood lipids in a randomized trial in men at risk of heart disease," Am L Clin Nutr (1994 May), 59:1060–8.

S Groziak et al. "Natural bioactive substances in milk and colostrum: effects on arterial blood pressure system," Brit J Nutr (2000), 84. Suppl. 1: S119–S25.

AH Lichtenstein et al., "Short-term consumption of a low-fat diet beneficially affects plasma lipid concentrations only when accompanied by weight loss," Arteriosclerosis and Thrombosis (1994 Nov), (11):1751–60.

GA Schoeller et al. "How much physical activity is needed to minimize weight gain in previously obese women?," Am J Clin Nutr (1997), 66: 551–6.

L Bartoshuk et al. "Effects of capsaicin densesitization on taste in humans," Physiology & Behavior (1991), 57(3):421–9.

LM Baroshuk et al., "Supertasting, earaches, and head injury: genetics and pathway alter our taste worlds, Neuroscience and Behavioral Reviews (1996), 20(1):79–87.

BH Tepper et al., "Fat Perception is Related to PROP Taster Status, Physiology & Behavior (1997), 61(6):949–54.

BJ Tepper et al., "Prop taster status is related to fat perception and preference," Annal of the New York Academy of Sciences (1998 Nov 30), 885:802–4.

A Hirsch, "What Flavor Is Your Personality?" Source Books, Inc., Illinois, 2001.

E Doucet et al., "Appetite after weight loss by energy restriction and a low-fat diet-exercise follow-up," International Journal of Obesity and Related Metabolic Disorders (2000 Jul 24), (7):906–14.

DS Hartman et al., "Diversity of dopamine receptors: new molecular and pharmacological developments," Polish Journal of Pharmacology (1997 Aug), 49(4):191–9.

G Gerra et al., "Neuroendocrine responses of healthy volunteers to 'techno-music': relationships with personality traits and emotional states," International Journal of Phsychophysiology (1998 Jan 1), 28(1):99–111.

J King, "Testing on the power of prayer," Science (1997), 276:1631.

P Wooten, "Humor: an antidote for stress," Holist Nurs Prac (1996), 10:49–56.

M Good, "Effects of relaxation and music on postoperative pain: a review," J Adv Nurs (1996), 24:905–14.

G Gerra et al., "Neurotransmitters, neuroendocrine correlates of sensation-seeking temperament in normal humans," Neuropsychobiology (1999 May), 39(4):207–13.

NA King et al., "Effects of short-term exercise on appetite responses in unrestrained females," Eur J Clin Nut (1996 Oct), 50(10):663–7.

"Tame Your Appetite," Health Magazine (2001 Jan/Feb), p. 115–120.

L Cruz et al., "Ingestion of chili pepper (capsicum annuum) reduces salicylate bioavailability after oral aspirin administration in the rat," Can J Phys and Pharm (1999 Jun), 77(6):441–6.

A Tremblay et al., "Increased resting metabolic rates and lipid oxidation on exercise-trained individuals: evidence for a role in beta adrenergic stimulation," Can J Physio and Pharm (1992), 70:1342–7.

T Watanabe et al., "Enhancement by capsaicin of energy metabolism in rats through the secretion of catecholamine from the adrenal medulla," Agriculture Biology and Chemistry (1987a), 51:75–79.

T Watanabe et al., "Capsaicin, the pungent principle of hot pepper, evokes catecholamine secretion from the adrenal medulla of anesthetized rats," Biochem and Biophys Res Comm (1987b), 142:259–64.

M Yosioka et al., "Effects of red pepper diet on energy metabolisms in men," J Nutr Sci Vitaminol 41:647–56.

K Takeuchi, et al., "Gastric motility in capsaicin-induced cytoprotection in the rat stomach," Jpn J Pharmacol (1991), 55:147–55.

Smart Choices

MW Gillman, et al., "Margarine intake and subsequent coronary heart disease in men," Epidemiology (1997 Mar); 8 (2): 144–9.

U Erasmus, *Fats That Heal Fats That Kill*, Alive Books (1993); 110.

INDEX

A
abdominal obesity, 17–18
achiote paste, 55
adobodo, 58
adrenaline, 37, 154
African "birds eye," 90
age, risk factor for heart disease, 34–35
alcaparrdo, 58
alcohol, 140–41
alder, 61
Allison, Heidi
    attempts to lose weight, xii–xiii
    designing Chili Pepper Diet, xiii–xvi
    diet that worked, 7
    health problems, xi–xii
American cuisine, reliance on fat, 8
American Heart Association, 4, 30
American Indian cultures, 27. *See also* Hopi
    culture
American restaurants, 224–25
Anaheim (chili), freezing, 78
ancho, 70–71, 87, 88, 107, 108, 111, 143, 146
    dried equivalents, 82
    heat of, 90
    powdered, 85
    starter chilies, 141, 145
    toasting, 83
ancho chili vinegar, 294
android obesity, 17–18
annatto seeds, 55
appetite suppressants, 5
apples, 47
applesauce, pureed, 49
arroz verde, 308
Asian cuisine, 8, 47
Atherosclerosis, 30

avocado leaves, 67

B
bagels, 127–28
baked goods, 49
baking, 50
balsamic vinegar, 52
banana leaves, 64, 67
bananas, pureed, 49
barbecuing, 60–61
basal metabolic rate, 119
bay leaf, 80
bell peppers, 46, 47, 89, 90
beta cell burnout, 20–21
beverages, 235–36
binges, tips for preventing, 150
bitter, 44
bitter lettuces, 52, 53
black mustard, 56
black pepper, 45, 56
black tea, 119
blood pressure, 25–26
blood sugar levels, 20–21
body mass index (BMI), 36
breads, 130, 199
breadspread recipes
    caper cream cheese spread, 249
    Chef Jamie Shannon's chipotle ketchup, 250
    olive cream cheese spread, 248
    savory poultry breadspreads, 251
    spicy Dijon spread, 247
breakfast cereals, 212
British Journal of Nutrition, 119
broth-based sauces, 49
Brownwell, Kelly, 4
buffets, 219

C

cabbage leaves, 64, 67
caffeine, 119
calcitonin gene-related peptide, 21
calcium, 137–39, 148–49
California (chili), 103
calorie counting, 3–4, 7
"calorie-free" foods, 185
calorie reduction, 114–15
canned beans, 201
canned green chilies, 143, 146
    avoiding with high blood pressure, 146
    heat of, 90
canned soups, 212
capsaicin, xiv–xv, 24, 88
    action with protein, 132–33
    activating pain receptors, 45
    asthmatics sensitive to, 142
    binding tightly to nerve receptors in mouth,
        148
    building tolerance to, 144
    causing vasodilation response, 15
    chemical makeup, 71–72
    development of, 72
    effect on brain, 12, 22
    effect on cardiovascular, digestive and
        immune systems, 15, 37
    effect on high blood pressure (hypertension),
        26
    effect on insulin, 21
    effect on liver and pancreas, 12
    effect on nervous system, 14–15
    exposure to, 72–74
    heat of, 89
    improving ability to process cholesterol and
        fats, 30
    improving circulation, 15, 141–42
    metabolic effects of, 8–9, 12
    pain-reducing properties of, 16–17
    physiological effects of, 13–17
    power of, 45–46
    similarities with nicotine on body's response
        to, 145
    source of heat in chili, 71
capsaicinoids, 71–72
Capsicum frutescens, 69
capsicums. *See* chili(es)
caramelizing, 59–60
carbohydrates, 4, 6
cardamom, 55, 56
Caribbean food, 231–32
cascabel, 70–71, 90, 109
casein, 148
cayenne, 99
    dried equivalents, 82
    heat of, 90
celery, 46, 47
central fat, 18–19
charcoal grilling, 62–63
cheese, 194–98
cherry (pepper), heat of, 90
chicken broth, 202
chicken stock, 50
chilaca chili, 108
chilaqil, 58

chili burn, putting out, 147–48
chili caballo, 93
Chili California, 104
Chili Colorado, 104
chili de àrbols
    dried equivalents, 82
    freezing, 78
    heat of, 90, 101, 144
chili equivalents, 146
chilies, 8, 9, 47, 55, 56, 56, 68
    alleviating stress, 37
    appetite suppressant, 23, 115, 141
    aroma enhancing flavor, 71
    augmenting beneficial effects of exercise, 32
    building tolerance to, 141–42, 143–44, 145
    buying dried, 81–82
    buying fresh, 74
    children and, 16
    classified as fruit, vegetable or spice, 69–70
    clinical study of dieting with, xv–xvi
    combining with garlic, onions, ginger,
        141–42
    controlling cravings, 27
    counteracting stress, 39
    decreasing absorption of aspirin, 143
    decreasing risk for heart disease, 33–34, 37,
        39
    depression-controlling effect, xv, 9, 33
    dieting without, 28–29
    difficulty in classifying, 69
    dried, 70–71, 81–85, 99–111
    drying, 78–80
    effect of adding to low-fat diet, 38
    effect on cholesterol, 37
    effect on glucose levels, 25
    effect on high blood sugar, 37
    effect on weight loss, 37
    endorphins released after eating, 17
    enhancing increase in metabolic rate, 119
    flavor linked to color, 70
    freezing, 77–78
    fresh, 92–97
    halting chocolate cravings, 28
    handling, 72–74
    in Hopi culture, 12
    hottest at lower branches, 71
    improving ability to process cholesterol and
        fats, 30
    improving taste of low-fat food, 8
    incorporating into diet, 143–46
    increased metabolic activity, xv, 22–23, 39
    increasing oxygen consumption rate, 39
    in low-fat vinaigrette, 52
    making paste from, 84–85
    measuring heat of, 88–90
    meat-flavored, 45
    methods of effecting weight loss, 22
    mirroring beneficial effects of exercise, 39
    missing ingredient in low-fat diets, 8–9, 24
    mixing red and green, 256
    nutritional content, 72
    oven-drying, 79–80
    peeling, 77
    picking, 80
    preserved in brine or vinegar, 85

preserving, 77–81
range of flavors, 70
reducing risk of diabetes and stroke, 34, 37, 39
rehydrating dried, 84
removing skin, 76–77
roasting, 70, 75–76
smoked, 45, 47
storing dried, 81–82
storing fresh, 74–75
sun-drying, 78–79
taking edge off dieting, xv
toasting dried, 83
tool for reducing fat, sugar and salt in diet, 88
use in different cultures, xiii
variations in location of "bite," 71
varying sensitivity to, 146–47
chili kachina, 12
Chili Pepper Diet
adding chilies to at least three meals per day, 125
alcohol, 140–41
breadspread recipes, 247–51
breakfast, 126–28
buffets, 219
calcium sources, 137–38
calcium supplements, 138–39
carbohydrate sources, 132
checking food labels for total fat, 184
cheese caveat, 198
chili consumption guidelines, 145–46
chilies, building tolerance to, 141–42
chilies, number of, 144
choosing goal weight, 151
control period, 28–29, 32–33
dessert recipes, 373–75
dinner, 128
effect on cholesterol levels, 30–31
egg recipes, 255–57
exercise, 155
fat intake, 122–23
fish consumption, 113–14
food shopping guide, 134–35
guidelines, 125
healthy fats in, 136–37
keeping fat budget, 149
kitchen tools suggested for, 119–21
lapses/relapses, 152–54
lunch, 128
maintenance plan, 123
margarine not used in, 205
marinade and sauce recipes, 341–45
meal plan, 122, 125
meat recipes, 315–17
one-day meal plan, 124
packaged foods, making smart choices with, 181–214
pasta recipes, 333–38
plateaus, 151–52
poultry recipes, 281–86
precautions, 142–43
proteins in, 132–33
realistic exercise regime with, 32
red meat, 137

reliance on serving sizes, 115
restaurant guidelines, 216–18
saboteurs, 152
salad dressing recipes, 271–77
salsa recipes, 349–61
science behind, 23–24
seafood recipes, 289–99
seasoning blend recipes, 365–70
serving sizes, 218
sides and salads recipes, 303–12
snacks, 128–29
soup recipes, 321–30
study, 28–29
style of eating, 115
supermarket guidelines, 182
supplements suggested, 148–49
twenty-one-day meal plan, 159–79
vegetarian recipes, 261–68
water consumption in, 139–40
weighing and measuring foods, 121–22
Chili Pepper Diet, recipes
breadspreads, 247–51
desserts, 373–75
eggs, 255–57
marinades and sauces, 341–45
meat, 315–317
pasta, 333–38
poultry, 281–86
salad dressings, 271–77
salsa, 349–61
seafood, 289–99
seasoning blend, 365–70
sides and salads, 303–12
soups, 321–30
vegetarian, 261–68
chili peppers, 43
chili pequeno, 100
chili peron, 93
chili powder, 47, 82, 85
chili rocoto, 93
chili seasonings, 210
chilitepin, 90, 100
chili vinegar, 52
Chinese (chili), 90
Chinese bamboo steamer, 67–68
Chinese food, guidelines for, 222–24
Chinese parsley. See cilantro
chipotle, 70–71, 87, 90, 105
chlorine, 139
chocolate binges, 27–28
cholecystokinin, 17, 325
cholesterol, xv, 4, 29–33, 35, 132, 136, 186
cider vinegar, 52
cilantro, 8, 55–56
cinnamon, 55, 56
citrus juice, 47, 53–54, 55
cloves, 55, 56, 148
cold smoking, 66
Columbus, Christopher, 9
Controlling Your Fat Tooth (Piscatella), 5
coriander, 56. See also cilantro
corn moth, 81
coronary artery disease, 29–30
cortisol, 27, 29
effect of elevated levels, 141

cortisol (continued)
  effect on fat storage, 18–19
  options for reducing, 19
cowboy beans, 306
cravings, 27
cream sauces, 48
Creole cuisine, 46
crushed red pepper flakes, 90, 145
cumin, 8, 55, 56
curry powder, 46–47, 56

D
dairy products, 137, 192–93
dark soy sauce, 51
deli food, 228–29
depression, xv, 4, 5, 9, 33, 114
dessert recipes
  spicy gingered pears with lemon cream,
      373–74
  strawberry gelato, 375
diabetes, 20–21
  risk factor for heart disease, 35
  risk related to type of obesity, 17–18
diet-induced thermic effect, 119
dihydrocapsaicin, 72
Dijon mustard, 47, 52, 54
distilled vinegar, 80
distilled water, 140
distilled white vinegar, 53
dopamine, 5, 28, 37, 114, 154
dried chilies, 55, 70–71, 145–46
dried poblano chili, 111
Dutch red chili, 95

E
Eades, Mary, 6, 7
Eades, Michael, 6, 7
eating, timing of, 116, 118
eating out, 5–6, 215–40
eating smaller meals, 115, 118
egg recipes
  breakfast burrito, 257
  eggs with mushrooms, onions and broccoli,
      255
  three-pepper omelet, 256
endorphins, 5, 17, 19, 22, 28, 88
en escabeche, 95
Epel, Elissa, 19
Erasmus, Udo, 187
estrogen, 35
European Journal of Clinical Nutrition, 9
exercise, 31, 114–15
  as appetite suppressant, 154
  boosting effects of, 37–39
  effect on weight and cholesterol, 36
  importance of warm-up and cool-down,
      155–56
  importance to diet, 154–56
  releasing endorphins, 19
  staying motivated, 156–58
"extra lean" foods, 184, 185

F
family history, risk factor for heart disease, 35

fast food, 234–35, 237–39
fat, American cuisine's reliance on, 8
fat-calorie ratio diets, 5
fat consumption, 4
fat cravings, 5
fat exchanges, 123
"fat-free" foods, 185
fats
  alleviating anxiety, 27
  flavoring food, 48
  hazardous, 133–36
  healthy, 133
  providing texture, 48
  replacing flavors when cooking without, 43
fennel, 61
fenugreek, 56
fermented pureed chilies, 85
fish, 202–4. See also seafood, shellfish listings
  grilling, 63–64
  role in diet, 114
fish oil, 114
flavor
  cooking for, 59–68
  importance of, 7–8
flavor combining, 43–44, 45–47
flavor marriage, 46–47
flavor opposition, 47
flavors
  primary, 46
  secondary, 46
food diary, 116, 117
food exchanges, 130–31
food labels
  checking serving sizes, 183–84
  interpreting terminology on, 184–86
  trans-fats not required to be listed, 186
Food Pyramid, 115
Francisca habanero, 89
frozen entrees, 188–90
frozen foods, 188
fruit, 47
  food exchanges, 130
  taste and enhancing flavor of, 129
fruit-flavored vinegar, 53
fruit spreads, 202
fruitwoods, 61
fruity wines, 50
"frying," nonfat, 50–51

G
garam marsala, 56–57
garlic, 45, 47, 50, 68, 80, 212
gas grilling, 63
German mustard, 54
Gillman, Mathew, 187
ginger, 8, 45–46, 47, 56, 57, 68, 212
gingerols, 45–46
glial cell line-derived neurotrophic factor, 16
glucose, 20–21, 25, 132
Goodfriend, Theodore, 26
grains
  creating texture, 48
  food exchanges, 130
Greek oregano, 57
green chilies, 70, 72, 75–76

green tea, 119, 226
grilling, 50, 62
    guidelines, 65–66
    preparing grill, 63–64
guajillo, 84, 106
    drying, 79
    heat of, 90
guëro, 96
gynecoid obesity, 18

H
habanero, 71, 87, 89, 90, 92
Hadjokas, Nicholas, 26
HDL cholesterol, 30–33, 35–36, 133, 136, 186
health-food stores, 183
heart disease, five controllable risk factors, 34–37
heart-healthy foods, 34
heart hunger, 153
heat, 88–90
Henry, C., 8, 119
herbs, 43, 45, 55–59
herb vinegar, 53
hickory, 61
high blood pressure, 145–46
high-pressure liquid chromatography, 89
high-protein diets, 6–7
Hirsch, Alan, 145
Holy Trinity
    chilies, 111
    Creole cuisine, 46–47
homodihydrocapsaicin, 72
honey mustard, 54
Hopi culture, 10–12
horseradish, 46, 54, 57
hot mustard, effect on metabolic rate, 119
hot sauces, 209
hot smoking, 66
"Hunan hand," 72–74
Hungarian paprika (hot), heat of, 90
hydrogenated fats, avoiding, 34
hydrogenated oils, 186
hypertension, 25–26

I
imitation crab, 204
Indian cuisine, 8, 55, 56, 58
Indian food, 233–34
Indonesian cuisine, 55
insulin, 6, 20–21
*International Journal of Obesity and Related
    Metabolic Disorders*, 30
iodized salt, 54
Iranian cuisine, 58
Italian food, 226–28

J
jalapeno, 71, 95, 145
    freezing, 78
    heat of, 90
    pickling, 80
Japanese food, 225–26
japones
    dried equivalents, 82
    freezing, 78

Journal of Clinical Endocrinology and Metabolism,
    137
juniper berries, 80

K
kachina dolls, 10–12
ketchup, 47
ketogenic diets, 4
Kiwon, L., 39
kosher salt, 51, 54–55, 80
Kristal, A., 8

L
LDL cholesterol, 30–33, 72, 132, 133, 136, 186
"lean" foods, 184, 185
legumes, pureed, 49
lemon, 47
lemongrass, 68
lemon juice, 53
"less fat" foods, 185
lettuce leaves (for preparing food), 64, 67
Lichtenstein, Alice, 7
"light" foods, 185
lime juice, 53
"lite" foods, 185
"low-calorie" foods, 186
low-fat cheese, 197
low-fat cooking methods
    dry, 60–66
    wet, 67–68
low-fat cuisine, improving, 43
low-fat diets, 4–6
    advocating exercise, 31
    chilies enhancing effects of, xv, 8–9, 22
    eating cheese in, 197–98
    meat in, 206–7
low-fat flavoring agents, 51–59
low-fat foods, xiii, 185
    improved with chilies, 8, 38
    lacking taste, 43
lycopene, 191

M
mace, 56
manzana, 93
maple, 61
margarine, 204–5
marinade and sauce recipes
    achiote citrus marinade (for roasted poultry),
        345–46
    savory meat marinade, 343
    smoky marinade, 342
    spicy citrus marinade, 341
    steamed vegetable sauce, 344
marinades, 210
mayonnaise, 208
meal plan, 159–79
meals, timing of, 142
meat
    as flavor, 45
    in low-fat diet, 206–7
meat recipes
    braised brisket with onion gravy, 315
    hamburger, 316–17

medium-tasters, 147
menopause, risk factor for heart disease, 35
mesquite, 45, 61
metabolism, xiv, 8–9, 12, 119
    alcohol's effect on, 140
    increasing, 22–23, 39, 118
Mexican cuisine, 8, 55, 56, 229–31
Mexican oregano, 57, 80
microwave popcorn, 212
microwaving, 67
Middle Eastern cuisine, 56
milk, most effective antidote for chili burn, 148
minced chives, 195
minced pickled peppers, 195
mirin, 47, 51
molasses, 47
mole, 46–47, 107
monounsaturated fats, 34, 136
morita, 90, 102
mouth surfing, 83
mulato, 111
    dried equivalents, 82
    heat of, 90
mushroom-flavored soy sauce, 51
mushrooms, 47
mustards, 43, 46, 54
mustard seed, 8, 57–58

N
nampla, 47, 51, 330
Nanami Togarshi, 226
National Cholesterol Education Program, 30
"natural" foods, 186
Natural Resources Defense Council, 139–40
nerve growth factor, 16
nerve plasticity, 15
nerves, function of, 14
neurotransmitters, 14
New England Journal of Medicine, 140
New Mexico (chili)
    drying, 79
    freezing, 78
    green, 103
    heat of, 90
    powdered, 85
    red, 104
nonfat cheese, 194–96
nonfat cooking sprays, 211–12, 214
nonfat "frying," 50–51
nonfat mayonnaise, 208
nontasters, 147
noradrenaline, 37, 154
nordihydrocapsaicin, 72
North African cuisine, 55, 56
"no sugar added" foods, 186

O
oak, 61
obesity
    abdominal, 17–18
    android, 17–18
    diabetes risk related to, 17–18
    dopamine levels related to, 5, 15
    gynecoid, 18
    health effects of, 3

linked to endorphin and neurotransmitter
    levels, xiv
oils
    providing texture, 48
    source of chili's fragrance, 71
oil sprays, 64
oily fish, 61
Old Bay seasoning, 68
oleoresin capsaican, avoiding, 142
olive oil, 52
omega-3 fatty acids, 114, 136
omega-3 oils, 202
onion, 46, 47, 50
orange habanero, heat of, 90
orange juice, 54
oregano, 55
Oriental cuisine, 55
osteoporosis, 235
Oxford Polytechnic Institute, 23, 119

P-Q
packaged foods, making smart choices, 181–214
pain, related to taste, 45
pan frying, 51
parsnips, substituting for cream, 48
partially hydrogenated fats, 133
partially hydrogenated oils, 186, 188
pasado, 71, 90, 110
pasilla, 97, 108, 111
    dried equivalents, 82
    heat of, 90
pasta recipes
    linguine in fresh tomato sauce with fennel
        and salmon, 336–37
    penne with roasted eggplant, tomato and
        kalamata olives, 333
    shrimp diablo, 338
    spaghetti alla Sicilian, 334–35
pasta sauces, 191–92
peperine, 45
peppercorns, 56, 80
pepperoncini peppers, 90, 143, 146
peppers. See chilies
pepper sauces, 85
pequin, 90, 100
phosphoric acid, 235
phytochemicals, 72, 308
pickled chilies
    limiting with high blood pressure, 146
    sulfites in, 142
pickled jalapenos, 95, 144
pickled peppers, 80
pineapple vinegar, 53
Piscatella, Joseph, Controlling Your Fat Tooth, 5
pizza, 200
poaching, 67
poblano, 70, 87, 97
    drying, 78
    freezing, 78
    heat of, 90
    method to avoid when removing skin, 76
polyunsaturated fats, 136
pomegranate, dried, 58
Ponzu sauce, 52
popcorn, 129, 212

portion sizes, focus on, 6
poultry, 205–6
poultry recipes
    Caribbean jerk chicken, 281
    Chinese chicken salad, 282–83
    Mexican chicken salad with avocado salsa, 286
    Mexican herbed poached chicken breast, 284
    soft chicken tacos, 285
powdered chili, 85
progesterone, 28
protein, food exchanges, 131
prunes, pureed, 49
pureed chilies, 85

R
radishes, 46
raisins, pureed, 49
Raven, Gerald, 7
recado, 58
red chilies, 70, 72, 79
red ginger, preserved in syrup, 276
red habanero, 90
red jalapeno, 95, 102, 105
red pepper
    effect on metabolism and appetite, 8–9
    nonpharmaceutical stimulant, 22
red poblano chili, 107
Red Savina habanero, 89, 90
red wines, 50
"reduced fat" foods, 185
reduction, 48
restaurants
    rules for dining in, 215–40
    serving sizes in, 215
rice, steamed, 49
rice wine vinegar, 8, 47, 53, 80
roasted chilies, 70
rocoto, 90
Rolls, Barbara, 126
rosemary, 45, 58, 61
Rutgers University, 147

S
sake, 52
salad-in-a-bag, 210–11
salad dressing, 200–201, 221–22
salad dressing recipes
    blue cheese dressing, 277
    creamy dill dressing, 274
    creamy light Caesar dressing, 271
    creamy tarragon dressing, 273
    sesame ginger salad dressing, 276
    spicy citrus dressing, 272
    spicy green chili salad dressing, 275
salads
    healthy, 220
    high-calories items, 221
    items to avoid, 220
    tips for, 220–21
salpimentado, 58
salsa, 209
salsa recipes
    avocado salsa, 361
    cilantro chutney, 356

fire-roasted salsa, 354–55
fresh tomatillo salsa, 349–50
red salsa, 357
roasted jalapeno salsa, 359
roasted salsa verde, 351–52
roasted serrano salsa, 360
salsa cruda, 353
salsa rojo, 358
salt, added to sugar, 47
salts, 54–55
salty, 44
salty/hot, 47
salty/tart, 47
"saturated fat-free" foods, 185
saturated fats, 34, 133
sauces, 48–49, 51–52
sautéing, 49–50
sauvignon blanc, 50
Scotch bonnet, heat of, 90
Scoville, Wilbur, 88–90
Scoville Organoleptic Test, 88–89
Scoville units, 89
seafood, grilling, 64
seafood recipes
    bagels with smoked salmon, caper cream cheese spread and tomatoes, 299
    broiled salmon with chipotle cream sauce, 289
    Chilean sea bass with tequila lime sauce, 292
    curried tuna salad, 298
    curried tuna sandwich, 296–97
    curry crusted trout, 293
    grilled swordfish with roasted pepper sauce, 290–91
    seared shrimp with ancho chilies, 294–95
seafoods. See fish, shellfish
Sears, Barry, 6, 7
sea salt, 55
seasoning blend recipes
    achiote paste (recado rojo), 370
    chili pepper diet recado (dry), 366–67
    smoky pasado chili seasoning blend, 365
    smoky recado paste, 368–69
seasoning pastes, 58
secret ingredients, 46
serotonin, 27, 28, 37, 154
serrano, 70, 94, 144
    drying, 78
    freezing, 78
    heat of, 90
    pickling, 80
serving sizes, 115–16, 129, 218
sex drive, 24
shallots, 52
shellfish, 47, 67, 203–4
sides and salads recipes
    broccoli slaw, 308
    charro beans, 306
    dry roasted curried potatoes, 303–4
    fresh corn with lime and chilies, 305
    refried black beans, 312
    rice verde, 310
    tabooleh, 309
    toasted Mexican-style rice, 307
    tropical fruit salad, 311

sleep, 29, 140–41
Slow Wave Sleep, 140–41
smell, related to taste, 44–45
smoked chilies, 45, 47
smoking, 66
soup, 49
soup recipes
    carrot soup, 329
    Chef Jamie Shannon's ancho chili eggplant
        soup, 327–28
    chicken congee, 330
    Indian orange lentil soup with ginger and
        garlic, 323–24
    smoky chipotle corn chowder, 321–22
    wild mushroom and barley soup, 325–26
soup and salad bars, 219–20
sour, 44
sour cream, 193–94
Southwestern American cuisine, 56
soy sauce, 8, 43, 47
special occasions, eating during, 239–40
spices, 55–59
spicy foods, personality and capacity for, 145
starches
    food exchanges, 130
    pureed, 49
steam frying, 68, 255
steaming, 67–68
stock, substituting for oils, 49–50
stress, 18–19, 27
stress fat, 17–19
stretching, 156
strong-flavored cheese, 197
substance P, 16, 73, 144
sulfites, 142
sumac, 58
sun-dried chilies, 145–46
supermarket guidelines, 182
super-tasters, 147
surimi, 204
Suter, Paolo, 140
sweet, 44
sweet/hot, 47
sweet rice wine, 47
sweet/salty, 47
sweet/sour, 47

T
Tabasco, 90
tamarind, 58
tarragon, 47, 52, 53, 68
taste
    biology of, 43
    related to aroma, 43–45
    relationship with pain, 45
taste buds, location of, 45
tastes, four elementary, 44
texture, 48
Thai (chili), 87
    dried equivalents, 82
    heat of, 90
Thai cuisine, 47, 51, 56, 232–33
thermogenesis, 22–23
thyme, 47, 58
tihu, 10–11

ti leaves, 67
tortilla, adding to soup, 49
trans-fats, 133–36, 186–87, 204–5
trigeminal nerves, 147
trigger foods, conquering, 149–51
triglycerides, 31–32, 34, 36, 114, 136
Tsili, 12
turmeric, 8, 56, 58–59

U
umami, 45
University of Memphis, 215–16
unsaturated fats, 136
unsweetened baby food, 49
U.S. paprika, heat of, 90

V
vacations, eating during, 240
vanilla, 44, 59
vasodilation, 15
veal stock, 50
vegetable-based cream sauce, 48
vegetables
    creating texture, 48
    food exchanges, 131
    grilling, 64
vegetable stock, 50
vegetarian recipes
    Cream of Wheat, 268
    goat cheese pizza with olives, 266
    oatmeal with cinnamon and blueberries, 267
    roasted poblano hummus, 262–63
    roasted red pepper and basil hummus, 264–65
    vegetarian burrito, 261
veggie burgers, 190–91
vinegars, 43, 52–53
vitamin A, 72, 191
vitamin C, 7, 72, 79

W-X
waist/hip ratio, 19
walking, benefits of, 154–55
water, 139–40
wax pepper, 96
white ginger, pureed, 276
white wine vinegar, 53
wine, substituting for oils, 49–50

Y
Yellow Hot Wax, 90

Z
Zewdie, Yayeh, 71